# THE LIFE OF HEATHER MAY

## Living with Recessive Dystrophic Epidermolysis Bullosa

WENDY SKERRY

Dedicated to H, Mel, Alex, Oliver, Amy, James and Jonny - as fragile as butterflies but with the courage of lions.

# What is Epidermolysis Bullosa?

EB is a genetic skin blistering condition. There are many variants and more are found regularly.

In general terms, the three main types are simplex, dystrophic and junctional.

Simplex, in general, is passed from generation to generation and affects hands and feet, causing blisters, which are painful and life-restricting.

Dystrophic, can be dominant or recessive. Recessive is a gene carried by both parents which means a 1:4 chance of the child being affected by EB. Unless they are aware that they carry the gene, the parents have no idea of the implications. The condition affects the outside and inside layers of skin, and can be mild or very severe; it is life-restricting and can be life-limiting.

Junctional, in general, is a gene carried by both parents, usually unknown by the parents. This type is so severe that children don't usually survive beyond their early years.

More information from DEBRA.org.uk

## What is RDEB?

Recessive Dystrophic Epidermolysis Bullosa. This is in layman's terms, so forgive me, professionals. It is a genetic condition which means that there are no anchoring fibres in the skin, any friction or blow causes the skin to blister or rip off leaving open wounds. Blisters have to be lanced as they travel and lift larger areas of skin. It affects the outside and inside of the body, also, the eyes, mouth and throat. Healing causes tightening and restriction of the skin. It can be life-restricting and limiting.

## DEBRA

Dystrophic Epidermolysis Bullosa Research Association. About forty-five years ago, a group of parents with children affected by DEB established this support group. Their main aim at this time was to fundraise and establish research to find a cure for DEB. When I joined DEBRA twelve years later, there was a paid director and an admin. support. The first Great Ormond Street Hospital EB specialist nurse had just been employed, funded by DEBRA, and the hope was for a cure in five years. Sadly, this proved to be a dream as realism showed that it was going to be far more complex in reality.

Since then, DEBRA has grown and is now a much larger organisation, supporting research and day-to-day living with EB, through fundraising, retail charity shops and patient and family support.

DEBRA is nationwide and worldwide. The aim is still for a cure and to no longer need DEBRA. Until then they continue to be mostly effective in their goals.

# Contents

# Prologue

I was once told that everyone has a book in them. I never believed this until now and my story is not fiction but that of my wonderful daughter.

But before I begin, let me tell you about my background. I was born and brought up in a lovely little village in Wiltshire. I had a loving mum and dad and a brother who I fell out with regularly, but love dearly. It was an ideal childhood, I went to the local primary school and secondary school in Marlborough, the local college in Swindon and then on to train to be a teacher in the Midlands.

I eventually got a job in Swindon and absolutely loved teaching. I progressed through my career and always thought that that was enough for me. I met and married my husband when I was nearly thirty and enjoyed life. However, the enjoyment was short-lived and we divorced after six years. I continued to enjoy life and my career and then met a man who was fun, but not for keeps!

However, surprise, surprise, I became pregnant and that's where Heather's story begins.

My reasons for writing this:

- I thought it might help with my grief. Sharing Heather's life would mean she is not forgotten in the future when my memories may begin to fade.
- An acknowledgement of what RDEB sufferers go through day in and day out, without complaint, and with a fierce determination to live. I know Heather (and I) found it difficult to understand suicide (a very controversial subject and I'm sure to get comments about this). But when your life is restricted in the way RDEB sufferers are and yet you still make the most of life, and enjoy every minute available, it's difficult to understand why you wouldn't want to continue to exist, especially as the ones left behind have their lives changed forever by suicide.
- I wanted to share how wonderful the NHS is. Over the thirty-plus years of being aware of EB, the NHS staff have become more and more supportive to the degree that they often refer to the parents/patients as experts, since they deal with day-to-day traumas. The next time you complain about having to wait twenty minutes longer for your appointment, remember, the staff are not sitting around having coffee, they are probably dealing with emergencies (which could be you one day). EB patients get used to being patient and waiting for vast numbers of appointments and often use their time creatively.
- Despite everything, over thirty-plus years, things have improved. There is now better maternity allowance time, job shares, access to education, and

yes, things can improve more, but they have moved on quickly in those years and we should celebrate these achievements.

- Finally, for all those who suffer grief whether it is EB connected or not. The two phrases you do not want to hear are: "You know where I am" and "Keep in touch". People grieving need others to reach out to them. Initially, a response from the grieving person may be short, but as time goes on, reaching out will help the person grieving to reconnect with the world.

- Note: apologies about the spelling of some of the dressings. I got used to using the dressings but not necessarily remembering how to spell the names. So many...

- I have deliberately not used the full names of people, only when it was essential. I'm not sure whether people would want their names in print, but I'm sure that each person would be able to identify themselves.

- My apologies to those who know, if I have got any of the details or events incorrect or in the wrong order. Trying to remember thirty years is quite a challenge.

- Finally, since writing this for my own benefit, I have decided to self-publish, perhaps it may help others and raise some funds for DEBRA.

# Pregnancy and birth (1990)

Apparently, I had an ideal pregnancy according to the nurse and midwife. I had no sickness, and I felt really healthy. By this time, I was acting deputy at a lovely school and looking to find a permanent deputy post, rather than return to my previous job, in a more challenging school, but one I loved.

To say the pregnancy was a shock is an understatement! I spent a long time considering options, adoption or whether I should keep the baby. Could I cope? My parents were amazing and were supportive of whatever I decided. Eventually, my maternal instincts kicked in: I would keep the baby. I can remember in February at five months pregnant, climbing up a ladder to put up hearts for our Valentine's celebration at school, and my boss went mad! But that's how well I felt.

My female friend came with me to all the maternity classes, we were probably both the oldest in the room. All the couples were in their twenties but I was thirty-seven. All my checks were fine, and so I prepared for the birth. I painted the nursery, yellow, blue, and grey, with Miffy pictures. No pink, I'm not keen on that colour, also no gender reveal! The cot and pram/pushchair were bought and assembled. And vast quantities of baby knitting were ready, made by me, Mum, Jackie, my cousin etc.

The Easter before the baby was due, my acting deputy role came to an end, and so I returned to my previous school. After Easter, I only had two weeks before maternity leave, as the baby was due on June 2nd (the day before my mum's birthday). We were due to attend a friend's wedding on the 1st, but I was convinced that I wouldn't make it; from the back, I looked ok, but the bump at the front was huge. It was three weeks until blast off!!

It was a very long three weeks. Since I was going back to work when the baby was three months old, at the beginning of September, I went into school to see my boss, to sort out which room I would have and which age group. I did actually have to go back two days before the end of term, however, because my maternity leave finished in the middle of the summer holidays, and because of that, I was deemed to be available for work!

I couldn't afford to stay off any longer as I had a mortgage to pay, and building societies were not very flexible in those days. I did consider job share, but in those days, it wasn't feasible unless there was another member of staff willing to job share, and at that time there was nobody (how things have changed). I had arranged child care with a very good friend, and my parents would have the baby on Mondays and overnight and take the baby to the childminder on Tuesday mornings so that I could go to my aerobics class on Monday evening and get a good night's sleep. All sorted!

I was on my way to see my friend during the three weeks and a girl drove out of a side turning and hit my car on the driver's side. Her dad came running out worried about her as she had only passed her test the week before. He failed to see that I was heavily pregnant (over eight months). Sadly, my little car "Tizzy", which was eleven years old and which I had had from new, was a write-off and I drove it onto the breakdown lorry. I got a payoff from the insurance company and a good friend who worked for Renault said he could get me a new car with a discount at the beginning of August. No worries, I could hardly get behind the wheel and I doubted I would be driving very far with a new baby. I wasn't hurt, but boy was I mad!

So now I was without a car and waiting... and waiting... I went to my friend's wedding, celebrated my mum's birthday, and eventually on the 13th (eleven days late) I went into labour

I started to have pains at 7.00 am on June 13th, went to the hospital and was assigned a lovely midwife. The midwife, I later found out, was on her first solo delivery. I was given to her as they didn't expect any complications. We met her in the lift at the hospital about seven years later, and she told us this. I said I was surprised she didn't give up there and then and she said it was a good learning curve. I also met her many years later after H's death, she said she had followed H's progress and had found her to be an inspiration.

H was born at 11.58 am. Apparently, I had the perfect labour – I'm really not sure that any mother would agree with that! But joy turned to worry very quickly. H was taken to the Special Care Baby Unit. I didn't see her until two hours later, and by then she had bandages on her hand and leg. They later showed me photos, her hand and leg looked like raw liver. At that time, we were one of the lucky ones. I heard stories of parents whose child was not diagnosed with EB until weeks later. I say lucky because one of the nurses working in SCBU thought she recognised the condition since a child had been born and taken there five years previously. And so, a dermatologist was sent for and she did a biopsy. A biopsy on a small baby. It was heartbreaking, but set me up for the trauma to come. DEBRA (Dystrophic Epidermolysis Bullosa Research

Association) was contacted and a newly appointed EB nurse from Great Ormond Street Hospital came down two days later to show us how to bandage.

At this stage, our first choice of a name for the baby was Alicia, which conjured up a little tiny baby. H was 8 lb 7 oz in weight and 52 cm long and looked like a mini sumo wrestler, with her layers of flesh! So, she became Heather May (May after my mother). And it suited her because she was like heather; a rugged plant that grows and flourishes in the toughest of conditions. Although, I have to say H never liked the name.

I stayed with H on the first night until 11.00 pm and then I was sent off to the mother and baby unit, which was tough as all the mothers had their babies with them, and so eventually I was put in a side room. The following day there was a stream of visitors, but only family was allowed, H's dad, my parents, and a series of women all claiming to be my sisters came to see me (I don't have sisters...) There was a short blond one, a short dark one, a tall redhead and one that drove from Brighton arriving at 8.00 am. She was allowed in because the nurses were kind, and then she cheekily asked for a cup of coffee.

Finding H a sleeping place was proving difficult. Initially, she was in an incubator – like Goldilocks, it was too small for her. Then the "goldfish bowl", but because she had so much padding, as advised by the EB nurse, she was perched on the top, so eventually they put her in a child's bed surrounded by bumpers and eventually silk sheets (my parents' friend worked for ICI and they sent us a ream to make into sheets). Again, this was recommended by the EB nurse. So, there she lay stretched out like a princess.

So, Isabelle (the EB nurse) arrived on Friday, two days after H was born. She showed us how to bandage, using vaseline gauze with hyoxile (not sure of spelling) gauze between fingers and toes, on her right hand and left foot, to stop the fusing, melolin cut into the right shape for the hand and foot, bandage and tubifast. The whole procedure took about an hour with a baby screaming at the same time.

Little did I know that at the time this was quick because as time went on, a baby begins to move and cause blisters which have to be lanced, and then have to be treated. Eventually, bathing, taking off old dressings and replacing them took up to two and a half hours. Also, until I put hyoxile on an open wound, I didn't realise how much it stung. This baby cried all the way through and I, and I am sure others, were left feeling the same as me, with ringing in the ears. But amazingly, I would pick H up under her bottom and neck (even as she got older, never under the arms as you could rip the skin off by causing friction) and cuddle her on her gamgee (cotton padding) to stop any friction, and within minutes after her initial sobs, she would be gurgling again.

With both hands and feet wrapped in bandages, because she had started getting blisters on the original unaffected hand and foot, we named her "teddy legs". Isabelle brought lots of pamphlets with her about EB and I read them all from cover to cover. Some gave me hope, others made me realise what an uphill struggle it would be.

The two pieces of information which stuck in my memory were that there was hope for a cure in five years, which has proved to be very optimistic; and that many RDEB sufferers only lived into early adulthood at that time. I hung onto the first piece of information that there would be a cure and therefore didn't need to worry about the life-limiting part.

I also bought from her a research manual, about 300 pages long. I read it and understood hardly any of it. I thought, perhaps, it would be best to live day to day and deal with issues as they occurred. At that time, I don't think I realised how many issues would occur. That was when I became a member of DEBRA.

The routine was established, I would wait for one of the nurses to be free and together we would do the dressings. She would hold H in the bath, I would soak off the old dressing, the nurse would hold her on her knee and I would put on the already prepared dressings. The preparation of dressings always gave me something to do while H was napping and within three days of H being born, I was doing dressings for my daughter, which I would do for the next twenty-nine years.

After a week the hospital decided they needed my bed! I went home every night at 9.00 pm and came back at 8.00 in the morning. I was expressing milk but H was finding difficulty in sucking, we soon realised that her tongue was becoming blistered. The first time I had to pop the blister on her tongue I was terrified. When H got teeth, she did it herself by biting on them.

The nurses came up with the idea of making the hole in the teat larger so that it could be literally poured down her throat! The wonderful men in maintenance did this for us.

Our daily routine became: feed H, then she slept, woke for dressings, cuddle and sleep, feed, go for a walk to Town Gardens using the dilapidated SCBU pram, back, feed, pop out while she was asleep to do admin or shopping, back, feed and settle her for the night. I guess I did eat during that time but my weight went down to seven and a half stones and at 5 feet 8 inches tall, I was pretty thin with no baby fat! I had food for the evening which Mum and Dad cooked and brought to my house, but I didn't always feel like eating.

But how did I get backwards and forwards, as my car had been written off? Well, when H's dad wasn't working he would drive me or let me have the car. But this became increasingly more difficult. My wonderful friend Jackie lent me hers and she walked to work. That's friendship for you.

One time I remember returning to settle H for the night and she was missing. I searched and eventually found her in the staffroom. All the other babies were mostly premature and slept a lot more and so were settled, but not H. She was wide awake and wanting attention, but the World Cup was on and England was playing, so all the staff wanted to watch it. She was in the staffroom being entertained while the staff watched the match. No wonder she always hated football.

We settled into our routine, always wondering when we could go home. Seeing premature babies leaving before us. The paediatric consultant insisted she drank two litres of milk per day before she went home, but this was rather a tall order considering it took her an hour to drink 125ml, and that was with large teats. Eventually, the dietician came up with the idea of mixing calogen and maxigel into the feeds to try and maintain her weight. This didn't work very effectively and she began to lose weight but still seemed very healthy. Eventually, I lost my temper and said that I was going to sign my baby over to the area healthy authority. Thank goodness for the senior nurse, Jo, in charge of paediatrics and therefore SCBU, who persuaded the consultant that she was better off at home, as I was already doing her dressings and the feeding might be better in a calm environment at home. I spent the next night in the mothers' room on the ward with H in a cot beside me. I can't remember sleeping much and was terrified of being on my own the next night, but determined that I could do it.

Five and a half weeks after H was born, we went home. I had to see the Chief Education Officer to give me my final two days as a leave of absence so that I could get paid. So, I then had six weeks with my baby but it was not all plain sailing. I went to school to show H to the staff and children, but obviously, they all wanted to hold her. Explaining that she had to be held on the gamgee (cotton layers, which were inserted into a pillowcase for padding), proved more difficult with the staff than with the children. This was probably because most of the staff were mothers and used to holding babies.

At home we were beginning to cope, dressings and feeding were always priorities, but evenings were an issue. The first time H screamed and brought her legs to her chest I was terrified. I phoned SCBU and they said that if I brought her up there, they may keep her in. There was no way I would do that, it took me long enough to get out!

I took her to my doctor, who also happened to have seen H at the hospital as she worked part-time in the paediatric department as well as being a GP. It was six-week colic and she taught me how to cope with it. Trying to hold H so that her legs didn't hit against me and cause blisters was the hardest thing, I felt like some kind of contortionist. Seeing my GP, we were also able to sort out the dressings and medicines I would need for a month and the pharmacy I would collect them from, since there were no deliveries then. Our doctor was wonderful and got us through those very difficult first years.

H's little pink book which I took to the baby clinic was an interesting read. She stayed firmly on the 70th percentile for height and gradually dropped from the 50th to the 20th for weight, despite everything I did. Luckily, the professionals told me not to worry, and thank goodness, it didn't drop further. We had to work very hard just to get enough milk into her to maintain her weight and keep her in the 20th percentile. Very soon I stopped taking the book with me.

The summer holiday was bittersweet since there was time to spend with H, but with the knowledge that there was so much organising to do, to make sure my childminder knew what to do. She came and spent sessions watching me do dressings and pierce blisters, she then did some – box ticked!

My wonderful Mum and Dad were busy making things secure, Mum, who was a wonderful seamstress, made bumpers, silk sheets, courtesy of our friend and ICI, covered the seams on clothes that couldn't be turned inside out, bought seamless baby grows from Marks & Spencer (M&S) (God bless M&S). My Dad secured all the above to cots, prams, and car seats. The first week at home, Mum and Dad helped with the dressings, until I could contact the community nurse to help me do the dressings.

I'd worked out that I could be home by 5.00 pm since school finished at 3.30 pm and then there were staff, year group meetings and preparation. But guess what, I couldn't have a community nurse after 4.30 pm. From all directions, I was being told that it was impossible to go back to work full-time and deal with an EB baby. All, except my lovely parents and friends.

So, we set in place a rota. Saturday evenings, I went to my parents, and they helped with the dressings, we stayed the night, had lunch on Sunday (always a treat), redid the dressings and had a walk around the village, stayed Sunday night, I went to work on Mondays leaving H with my parents and they did her dressings.

I went home on Monday evenings, stayed late at school after the staff meeting to get as much done as possible and then went to aerobics. Tuesdays I went to school and my parents dropped H at the childminders. As she got older, they used to go via Toys 'R' Us (buying all sorts of presents – thank goodness we had a playroom). They were remarkable people considering they were in their seventies.

I would collect H from the childminder, Aunty Jackie and Uncle Bob would come and do dressings and we would eat together – me cooking one week and Jackie the next (Jackie's "chicken thing" was always a favourite). As H got older, she would have a sip of beer with Bob or wine with Jackie and I. She rarely had pain relief for the dressings but the sip of booze put her in a good mood! Wednesdays were spent with Aunty Flo Jo and a beer, and Thursdays were spent with Aunty Pat and sherry.

Heather's dad occasionally did Thursdays but shift work meant he was less reliable to be there every Thursday. When H reached six months, we went swimming on a Thursday with Aunty Pat at the local hydrotherapy pool. We both went in the water with H, Pat would get dressed, I would bring H out of the water and quickly get dressed and then do H's dressings in the medical room at the hydro. They were brilliant people, so caring and flexible. Friday was always an issue, with it being the weekend, until Aunty Jackie J stepped up to the mark. She was driving and so we had tea, coffee or a soft drink. My week was covered.

The other issue was that H was reluctant to go to the toilet, and had a fissure in her back passage. This meant that when she looked as though she wanted to go to the toilet, she would often cross her legs to stop herself from going, we had to force her legs open, which often caused more friction and damage, but we achieved it and eventually, she began to realise that it was better to go and hurt a little rather than wait until the stool became, as my mother said, the size of a big dog! The lactulose she was given worked to a degree, but the toilet issue went on for about two years.

The first time I was really aware of H's fragility was when she was still in hospital and I changed her nappy. The tape had stuck to her skin and I panicked, instead of asking for help, I ripped it off like a plaster and took three inches of skin with it. I dressed it as best I could but then it got infected and she had to have antibiotic cream on it. You can imagine the profound effect it had as I can still remember it to this day – thirty-plus years later.

We also had to give up on putting dressings between the toes, since trying to hold a baby's leg when they move it up and down was challenging, and we were doing more harm to the back of the leg. This meant that her toes fused on that one foot, which wasn't too much of an issue when she was little, as we were able to pad her shoes, but as she got older there was a considerable difference in size and so we had to buy two pairs of the same shoes, always making sure we threw away the correct shoe for each size! Such a waste. We tried through shoe companies to find others with the same but reverse problem, so that we could give away the spare shoes, but had no luck.

Before walking, H crawled, but I use the term loosely, with a damaged leg and hand, she looked more like the "Hunchback of Notre Dame". She damaged herself a little, but nowhere near as much as when she started to walk, which wasn't unaided until she was nearly two. When a toddler falls over, the knees and hands are usually damaged, but with H it meant constant knee and hand dressings. Riding a bike was even more challenging, although she didn't persevere with this for very long.

Her fingers and toenails gradually fell off, and as with teeth, after the tooth fairy had finished with them, I kept them all. When I told H she was disgusted! We were very lucky that her face was almost unaffected except when she was a small baby and rubbed her face when she was tired. In fact, as she got older, she made more fuss when she had a "zit'" than any wounds, and would insist that because I had nails, I squeezed them. I found this disgusting!

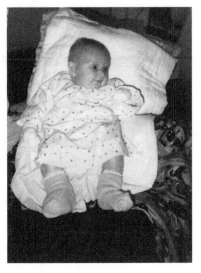

Teddy feet.

## 2

# Pre-school (1990-93)

From September, life settled into a pattern. The more H moved, the more blisters occurred, despite padding everywhere including clothes, this meant more dressings and a varying dressing routine each night. But everyone coped well, and preparing the dressings before helpers arrived, meant bath and dressings only took between one and a half hours and two hours.

As time went on the dressing regime changed, advice from our nurses meant no longer having to use a template for the leg and cut out the melolin, we ditched the Vaseline gauze and hyoxile and started to use mepitel, lyofoam for padding and secured it all with the tubifast. We found this gave H more flexibility in her limbs.

Individual quality time for H and I was limited to nights, first thing in the morning and weekends, but we coped. In general, after dressings and food, people went home at about 8.30 pm, just after H had fallen asleep, I would put her to bed and then do about two hours of school work, prepare for the morning and get ready for bed. She would wake for a feed at about midnight and then hopefully (not always) sleep until 5.00 am. If she was uncomfortable or a blister occurred, she would wake screaming and then take a while to settle. At 5.00 am I fed and changed her and then did the ironing and got myself ready for work.

Luckily, I had a cleaner and so I didn't have to worry too much about the house. Off we went to the childminders at 8.00 am. There was no time to think about H during the day, although I did, as I had a class of thirty seven-year-olds to deal with. I couldn't check on her, as we had no mobile phones back then.

H was baptised in October half-term, or as one child said at the baptism, "capsized"! Jackie and Bob and Flo and Mac were her godparents and I couldn't have wished for better people to help her through the first few years. My mum sorted and mended the family robe, the one that David and I had both worn and H had a white fur jacket. She looked lovely, and then she got fractious and rubbed her head, taking off a layer of skin and so she then had to wear a white headband dressing. If she'd had hair she would have looked like a hippy.

Then came the bombshell, I was aware that the childminder had taken on more work, cleaning for some elderly people, which meant taking H with her. Initially, I was OK with it, but then there were issues with her dressings. The childminder decided it was too much and gave me notice, to take effect from after Christmas. My parents said they would drive from the village every day but this was only a short-term solution. Up stepped the wonderful "earth mother", Boz, my friend from college when we were sixteen. Boz took her in, cared for and nurtured her and gave her two "brothers" who she adored.

In fact, Boz is of Polish descent and so H's first words were Polish.

Boz was the perfect person for the process of feeding; at the time, we didn't realise that H had a restricted oesophagus, and Boz spent hours at the weening stage persuading her to eat, liquidising her food to make it easier to swallow. Sometimes there was little time between meals. So not only did she have a very comfortable time, the attention of two lovely boys, Boz and the lovely Kais, who referred to her as "Habibi'" (Arabic and Polish!). What could go wrong? H's speech developed rapidly, understandably more quickly than her physical development. In fact, on her second Christmas when we took her to meet Santa on a train, she was able to glare at him and say: "Get off me!" - nice!

Our first trip to Great Ormond Street was in October when H was four months old. Heather's dad drove and my mum came with us, little did I realise that the trip would become familiar and I soon would be driving us up to London. When we arrived at GOSH we must have looked like we had come for the week. Not only did I bring medical supplies and clothes, but we also carried H's bath, so that I could bathe her and soak off the old dressings, before applying the new ones. It never occurred to me that we were in a Children's Hospital. Duhhh!!

We met the wonderful Professor Harper (our consultant), and Jackie, who replaced the first EB nurse we had. Jackie stayed with the EB families for many years, she was a font of knowledge and a great support, realistic and practical. Lesley, our amazing dietician, Michelle, the physiotherapist, who H loved over the years she knew her and they spent a lot of time laughing together, the occupational therapist and many other people. We were there at 10.00 am and didn't leave until 5.00 pm, but I felt as though I knew a little more about what I was facing.

I didn't realise at the time that the multi-disciplinary team had not been established for very long, and it certainly took the pressure off seeing different professionals at different times. From then on, we routinely went to GOSH every six months and they always tried to fit it into holiday time, so that I didn't have to take time off work. It didn't always work, but the Headteacher and Governors of the school were very understanding. We also had six monthly visits to our local hospital to see the dermatologist who did the biopsy, and after she retired, we had another lovely lady, who was our dermatologist until the end. Amazingly, later when H was in her teens and transferred to St Thomas' Hospital, our EB consultant knew our dermatologist at the local hospital. In fact, they did their training together. I guess it's a small dermatology world. We were seen by a variety of professionals every three months.

Our first Christmas was spent with Mum and Dad, and Boxing Day with Flo and Mac, Mum and Dad. The pressure was off and I spent a lot of time sleeping. So did H which made it difficult to open all her presents, and boy did she have a lot of presents. Flo made her a cuddly octopus (Olivia Octopussy), which she could lie against and was padded and well supported. Mum and Dad bought her an indoor swing, with a padded seat and padded straps.

January came too quickly and we settled back into a routine. Heather's dad had his own flat but spent much of the time with us when he wasn't working a shift. He had a first-year student nurse living in the flat below him, and in her "wisdom" she told him that the EB couldn't be an affected gene on both sides, as he already had a son who wasn't affected. Obviously, she knew more than the EB professionals. It was pointless playing the blame game as it didn't help with day-to-day care.

Eventually, when H was about six months, we decided that I would bring H up, he would have contact and pay maintenance. The maintenance paid for half the childminding. He would see H on a Thursday unless he was working and then we would arrange another day. The only problem was that there were always people there helping with the dressings, and it was quite difficult to ask them to leave. They had helped with dressings, gone through the trauma of the crying, with there being less screaming as she got older and could be entertained, and it didn't seem fair for them not to get the pleasure of a happy baby now. Gradually, his visits became more ad hoc, although he always kept in touch.

H's birthdays were always a great event. From her first birthday, with lots of children and adults until her eighteenth and twenty-first, there was always a party and her birthday celebrations usually went on for several weeks. She loved a good celebration.

In the summer of 1991, after the first Iraq confrontations began, Boz and Kais brought his parents over from Iraq. It was impossible for Boz to deal with everything. Although she was reluctant, it made sense for me to find another childminder. This time it wasn't quite so difficult, and I found a lovely mum with children at our school, who coped with everything. H had time with her during the summer holidays and had then acquired two "sisters". Karen looked after H for two years, until she was three, taking her to mother and toddler groups and then playgroups. Then she got remarried and moved away.

Just before the summer holidays, when she was one. H stopped drinking and eating, and she had to be admitted to the hospital and was put on a drip to rehydrate. This was the first of many traumatic incidents, but it made me grateful for our wonderful NHS.

We had our first summer holiday away with Mum and Dad in a cottage in Devon. It was a relief to be away and such a joy to be with H. The following year we went with Mac and Flo, Mum and Dad to Wales to another cottage. By then H loved swings and there was a rocking swing in the garden. Well padded, H sat on one side and Mac (over six feet tall) sat on the other side with his knees up to his neck.

When H was two, Mum and I decided to take her to Spain to meet my brother, who hadn't yet seen her. Dad stayed at home with the dog. The journey was very smooth, partly because I went to my local independent travel agent, who took all the details, and arranged everything from early boarding, an extra allowance for baggage, dressings etc, and the facility to take the medical kit with me on board, with needles in for piercing blisters and medicines. It made life so much easier. From then on, I used her, she was an amazing lady, who kept all the details, so I never had to worry. My brother collected us from the airport. He was enamoured, if a little scared, by this cheeky little 2-year-old, still dodgy on her feet, but with an extensive vocabulary. This became a life-long friendship and love between H and her Uncle Dai (David).

While we were there, he and his partner took us to a wildlife park. There was an elephant in an enclosure and we went to see him after getting an ice cream. H was in her pushchair and the elephant came close, managed to put his trunk over the low wall and scoop the ice cream out of her hand. He was very gentle, there was no damage, just surprise. She didn't cry but put her hand out because she wanted to stroke him. This was the beginning of her lifelong love of elephants. Despite a high UV level of suncream, H managed to come back looking healthy, and not burnt. This helped her to be sensible, during all her holidays.

Also, around this time, we began to see that H had a problem with her eyes. We saw a lovely consultant at GOSH as well as one at our local hospital who recommended drops and later on, really cool tinted glasses. This didn't stop her from getting blisters in her eyes which was more debilitating than the dressings sometimes, and meant she had to lie down and close her eyes until the pain was less. Another place we have skin.

H was about two and a half when we decided to set up a DEBRA fundraising group. Jackie had organised sponsored aerobics soon after H was born and the money raised from that went to SCBU. Now she set about arranging another session, but this time it was going to be bigger and better, so we needed a committee: Jackie and her new partner Rob, Jackie and Rich, Adelaide, Pat, Lorraine and myself (with help from H). It was an amazing success raising over £2000. School friends and colleagues, ladies from Jackie's aerobics class, and many others came.

From then on, we did fundraising events every three months. We held one big one each year and three smaller ones. We had a proper committee and help from David at DEBRA. For thirteen years we carried on with this system, and during that time we froze collecting outside Toys 'R' Us; collected at the "dogs", which H loved as Rob put on a bet for her and she won; "Fool in the Pool" – the manager of the hydrotherapy pool opened specially on a Sunday for us free of charge, we all dressed up, played games and had damaged ears from all the children screaming; a golf tournament, arranged by Adelaide, using her influence as a Councillor to get the Mayor involved; collecting at an event at Lyneham (courtesy of Flo and Mac); 50/50 club, run by Jackie J at school and based on the bonus ball on the lottery; a sponsored haircut by a wonderful man who had long hair all the way down his back and agreed to have it shaved off for sponsorship, he was also a member of the local bikers group, so that was a brilliant evening etc, etc. The people involved were amazing, and all those who contributed money, over a thirteen-year period, were also amazing.

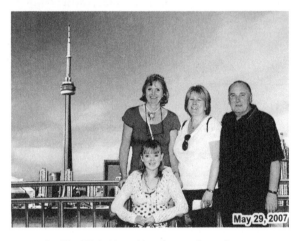

May 29, 2007

Jackie, Rich H and I - always there for us.

Over the years, many people raised money for DEBRA after meeting H. Including five very enthusiastic people who did the three peaks challenge (Scafell, Snowdon and Ben Nevis) over a weekend, as they all had to go to work on the Monday. Another event was when a friend did a parachute jump for a special birthday and instead of presents, asked for money for fundraising.

H and I being on our own had its challenges, especially when she was very young. Anyone with a small baby knows that getting a shower can be difficult. I always took H into the bathroom with me. That was fine until she could crawl, and for some reason, she felt it important that I should always have my slippers in the shower. So many pairs of wet slippers. As time went on though, we became a team. She would help where she could, emptying the small bins in each room, doing a bit of dusting, and when I fell from a ladder painting the hall, she got the frozen peas from the freezer and phoned a friend to take me to A & E. Nothing was broken, thank goodness.

# 3

## Going into school (1993 onwards)

After Karen, I was lucky enough to get the wonderful Lorraine. Like Karen, she was also a parent in the school but had more recently become a dinner lady (MDSA) and Teaching Assistant (TA). This was when future planning and my access to education became useful.

It was agreed that Lorraine would continue as a TA on Mondays, when H was with Mum and Dad, and Lorraine would continue working in school to keep her contract open, with the understanding that when H came into school Lorraine would be her 1:1.

The Local Education Authority (LEA) agreed that she could come to the school where I worked, even though officially she was out of the catchment area. I had support from the Head and the Governors, and because, by then, I was the Special Needs Coordinator, I was able to know the right route to access the PASSIS team (physical and sensory support team).

The wonderful Mary came and sorted a medical room with a table and storage for H's dressings, paid for by the authority and most useful to the school even after H left the school, and generally looked at issues around the school.

I applied through the LEA special needs department for a Statutory Assessment of Educational Special Needs (Statement), and our wonderful Educational Psychologist came to visit and assess the situation. Bless him, he was mostly used to dealing with children with learning difficulties and so when H completed his wooden shape puzzle in seconds, he gave up on the cognitive and concentrated on the physical. Unfortunately, he lost a piece of his very old wooden puzzle and phoned me at regular intervals to ask if I had found it. I searched the house and he obviously had lost it elsewhere, probably in his very untidy car.

The Statement came through before H started school and with it, money to pay for Lorraine also came through. Mum and Dad weaved their usual magic and padded everything she would use in the school, including her school uniform. I wrote a simple book for the class explaining her condition and Jackie J illustrated it. This was used during her infant school life.

All was set to go, and in the time before H started school, she enjoyed her time with her new family. This time two boys and a girl. She went to playgroup with Lorraine and there she met her life-long friend, Nik. Nik went into nursery, but H couldn't as she was out of the catchment area. They reconnected, however, when they started school, the term before they were five, in a friends' class. It was a large class of over thirty children, which had gradually grown in size over the year, with an intake every term. Because of this she only had one term in reception which went very quickly.

By the time H had reached two, she was more able to help with dressings and so, in general, we did them on our own, although we still had company from our friends, which involved more play than medical procedures.

She still liked people coming to help with the dressings, especially if she could spread the Diprobase cream over faces as well as herself. I had to warm the Diprobase as in her opinion it was too cold, and poor Jackie J had to have it spread on her face by H to make sure it was the right temperature. H's leg and hand had healed, although they were scarred, and one leg was thinner than the other. But with movement, she was causing more blisters and skin to be ripped off causing her to need dressings in other places. The medical room at school was a bonus because it meant that any problems could be dealt with immediately. It took a while for me not to interfere, but luckily, I was "locked" in my own room with my class. I rarely got sent for, as they all coped so well.

When H was three, we were invited with other DEBRA families to a Christmas party at Harrods. I don't think I've ever seen so many excited, uncontrollable children in one room. Mum, Flo, H and I found a quiet table and saw the entertainment, had vast quantities of food, lovely presents, and then Mr Blobby arrived, falling all over the children and heading our way. I stood up to protect H and luckily, he missed our table, but unluckily he fell over my foot!

I don't think anyone noticed as he just bounced from place to place anyway. At the same party, a famous celebrity picked up one of our EB children under the arms, before the mother could stop him. The child didn't react until after he left, and then the mother had lots of underarm dressings to do. Our EB kids are so resilient, but accidents happen so quickly, no matter how careful you are.

Mum and Dad sold their house in the lovely village and moved to Swindon, just so they could be close to us and help out. We still went back to the village, mostly so that we could play Pooh Sticks at the river.

H moved into year one with another lovely teacher. She began going to the hydrotherapy pool with the school, as some PE was rather challenging. She could manage the low apparatus but climbing frames and ropes caused too much friction. She loved to dance and to use the small apparatus. She went swimming and caught up with her school work when the others did types of PE that she couldn't join in with.

I decided that getting her a small trampoline for her birthday would help strengthen her legs and arms. It was one that had a bar to hold on to. I collected it and stored it upstairs in the spare room. H was staying with Mum and Dad one evening and I had gone to aerobics. When I got back, I locked the door, and put the bath on, which was downstairs and took an age to fill. I went upstairs and put the trampoline together, lifted it, and got it stuck on the stairs, with me behind it. The bath was still running... Luckily, I had a phone upstairs (pre-mobile phones), so I phoned Lorraine, she sent Pete with a key, switched off the bath and got the trampoline downstairs. Oh, thank goodness for good friends. H loved the trampoline.

Mum and Dad bought her a "Wendy House" which she loved and spent hours in. Gradually it became too small for her, and one day she banged her back on it damaging herself quite badly, she was so reluctant to get rid of it that we bought her a full-sized shed, which Jackie J decorated in purple, pasted with recycled CDs and hung a beaded curtain. It was amazing and no longer looked like a shed. She and her friends used it for many happy years.

Going to the hydro during school time meant that she didn't go on Thursdays, but Aunty Pat still came to tea. Lorraine changed H's dressings when they went swimming and another wonderful TA would often help her, she named H

"'Socks'" as H would wear two pairs of socks. One inside out to stop rubbing and one the right way around, which also gave extra padding.

Parents' evenings were always interesting, although my colleagues were always honest. H saw school as more of a social event than anything else, especially when she was in year 2.

Lunchtime was challenging as H ate very slowly but also wanted time with her friends. She was used to grazing during the day which kept her weight up, but this wasn't possible in school. I was suddenly aware of her size compared to others when she wore her aerobics outfit at one of our many fundraising events. It was pink and purple shorts and a crop top. I could see every rib, and her arms and legs looked so thin.

On our next visit to GOSH, we discussed it with Jackie and Lesley. We had tried giving her build-up drinks, but H hated them, and said they were thick and gritty. It was decided to give her a Barium Swallow Test to see where the problem was. Her throat was like an egg timer, which narrowed, making it difficult to swallow and making her feel full up. A gastrostomy tube was suggested and it was explained to us and we were given literature. I don't think I've ever had so many sleepless nights thinking about something. Putting a foreign body into your child and all the things that could go wrong with it. But I was also aware that any nutrition was going into the healing process and not into growth.

When she was five, she had a gastrostomy peg fitted. When your child is being operated on, that's when you feel useless and time drags. It was also the time we found out that she had a very bad reaction to the anaesthetic. She was being sick, despite the anti-sickness medication, but the button (peg) was in place.

We kept it clean and eventually began feeding H overnight, with what I can only describe as something like neat cream, but with a strange smell.

The pump we had that administered the feeds was quite noisy, but we got used to it. We were told that the peg would need changing about every six months unless the balloon burst. The balloon held the button in place and the water had to be changed every week. The first button change was done by the community nurse, and from then on, we did it. We settled into a good routine and everything went well until I tried to change the water one weekend and nothing happened, we were convinced that the water was still in as the button was firmly in situ. We tried to push the valve but with no success.

On the following Monday, I phoned the community nurse and she came out to school. My boss kindly took my class, and H, Lorraine, the nurse and myself crammed ourselves into the medical room. I explained that I thought there was still water in the valve, but she was insistent that the button just needed a good tug. I pointed out that it wasn't loose, and still flush to the skin. Before I could say anymore, she pulled the button and the balloon was still inflated, luckily there wasn't too much blood, but H was distraught and in great pain. Needless to say, from then on H was reluctant to have her button changed, and two of us used to battle with her for an hour, with her screaming and swearing, back to the ringing in the ears. Afterwards, a very large glass of wine was needed for me!

As time went on, H started to take the button out herself when it was due to be changed. The sight of her relief when the 5 ml came out through the valve, then an hour while she gradually took the old one out, and put a new one in was wonderful. I used to make dinner while she was replacing the button. Despite this trauma, it was still the best decision I made. It took away the pressure of eating and meals became fun and a social event. In fact, as time went on, going out for dinner was one of her favourite activities.

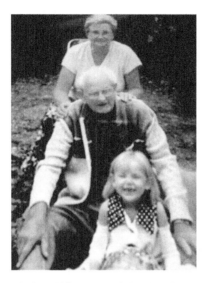

mum, dad and H on one of their lovely picnics.

H put on a lot of weight quite quickly, and at one point I was concerned that it was too much. I phoned the dietician and left a voicemail saying that I thought H was getting chunky. Lesley phoned back later in the day and left me a voicemail recommending leaving the calogen out of the overnight feed as it had only been added to the feeds to improve her weight, then hopefully she would be less chunky. Unfortunately, H heard the message and was less than impressed that I had called her chunky. A great deal of grovelling had to be done.

She kept her button from then on, it was like a safety blanket. When she was struggling to eat or we were in a hurry we knew that she had the goodies required for healing and growth. The only downside was that occasionally the pump would leak and that was like having neat cream poured onto a carpet, so we soon learnt to cover every area just in case.

4

# The junior school (1997-2001)

The transfer to the junior school was less traumatic than I expected. The whole time she was there she had brilliant teachers. The first one made a book, with her then-existing class, with questions for H to answer. It was a wonderful way to break the ice and make the whole school aware of her condition. The other plus was that Lorraine transferred with her, as the Headteacher agreed it was quicker, easier and safer to have someone who knew what she was doing.

The Local Education Authority also converted a medical room under the supervision of our expert. She loved junior school, mostly I suspect because she was totally away from me. She joined the Brownies, took part in the disabled swimming tournament, swam for Wiltshire and came first. That was a proud mummy moment. She also played the recorder – enough said. It was around that time that we realised how flexible she was when she was able to get her legs around the back of her neck.

During her time in junior school, we continued to go to GOSH, and on one visit Michelle the physiotherapist took us to the pool and took photos which were made into a book to help other EB patients with swimming exercises. I think it took a lot longer than it should have as there was a great deal of giggling and chatting.

She was also involved in the Butterfly Launch:

"The skin is as fragile as a butterfly's wings"

It's the symbol of DEBRA to this day. Through this, we became involved with Luke who ran the butterfly house at our local garden centre. A fascinating place and they did lots of fundraising for DEBRA.

We also made the papers for a totally different reason. I had bought Heather a large inflatable plastic ball which she could lie on and gave her movement as we moved her around the garden. It helped her coordination and balance. One evening it accidentally got left in the garden instead of being put away and was stolen. Somehow the local paper heard the story and did an article, then the nationals got hold of the story too. One of them bought her a replacement ball but most of all it was great publicity for EB and DEBRA. I always remember the photo of H holding the ball above her head. Impossible! It certainly was, what nobody could see was Lorraine and I holding the ball and H just touching it.

We appeared in the Life Line appeal. Travelling up to Worcester to meet another EB girl, who was younger than H. The filming was with Tom Conti. I was so excited and chatted to H all the way up about his career and what a wonderful actor he was. The filming took place in a local park, and as we went up the path, I pointed Tom out to H. To which she replied: "He's old!" I was gutted, how could she say that? However, he won her over with his natural charm.

On another occasion when she was in junior school, she was invited to go to RAF Lyneham and meet Princess Anne. It was near the end of the summer term, and we had managed that year to have all hospital appointments out of school time, and no illnesses or time off. So, she would get her 100% attendance and a trip out with the other 100% attendees. She wrote a letter explaining this and refused the invitation, and received a lovely letter back from the Princess Royal. I still wonder if it had been Prince William would she still have refused?

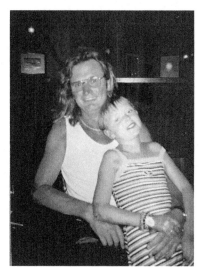

Uncle Dai with H.

The local Cubs/Scouts also did fundraising for DEBRA. I still have a lovely cutting of H and the cubs/scouts, one of whom was Waylon who went on to star in musicals in the West End, and H followed his progress with pride. Over the years many organisations have been touched by the EB condition and raised funds for DEBRA, from a gymnastics club to a ladies' choir.

On another of our visits to GOSH, Amanda Holden was due to visit a cancer patient but unfortunately, the child wasn't well enough for the visit, so she came to see the EB patients, H was enraptured by her and Amanda spent ages sitting on H's bed talking about makeup, pop stars and strangely H was fascinated by Amanda's nail varnish, which considering H didn't have any nails was very interesting. What a lovely lady. H loved seeing her on *Britain's Got Talent*.

She was less impressed when she was given a signed CD of Gary Barlow's first solo song after Take That split up. H was rather young for Take That, and so didn't appreciate it. In later years I constantly reminded her that she gave it away.

H's junior days were probably the least traumatic, that's not to say that problems did not occur, but I guess we dealt with them.

5

# Holidays

Holidays in Britain were always much easier than going abroad. Usually, because we could pack up the car and there was always a pharmacy close by. Although, apart from Calpol, I can't really remember the need to use them, but there was always that security in having them, as well as easily being able to contact EB nurses.

Devon, Cornwall, Wales and the Lake District were always favourites, mostly with Mum and Dad. When H was about four years old, DEBRA bought a caravan in Weymouth and sited it at Bowleaze Cove, this then became our happy place. We were one of the first visitors to the new caravan and it was absolutely lovely, and spacious, with fans to keep us cool, and a wonderful body dryer in the wet room, which we all took advantage of. I can't remember how many times we went there, but it was usually once or twice a year with different people, Mum and Dad, Lorraine and family, Jane and Becky and then later on, H would go for girly weekends with her friends.

When she was very little, the cup and saucers ride was a favourite and Bret who worked on the fair would often forget to get her off and so she would have two or three rides for the price of one. We got to know the people there and the lady in the booth got very used to exchanging H's pocket money for 2p pieces to spend on the 'Tipping Point machine'. I used to leave H and Mum there and go for a coffee. They would spend up to an hour on it and usually come back with a profit.

We spent one holiday there for my birthday with several friends which involved a lovely Italian meal, vast quantities of wine and going down the Helter Skelter. I don't think H was impressed by my behaviour and I wasn't impressed by my hangover. More holiday homes were added and we had breaks in Poole, Blackpool, Scotland and the Lake District. There was even one in Brittany, where Lorraine and family, H and I had a lovely holiday.

One of our holidays at the caravan was a bit of a disaster, we had gone with H's godchildren and were enjoying a day trip to a village which had been used during the Second World War for manoeuvres and so the villagers had to leave and they did not return. The village was still left as it had been in the 1940s period. The village was low in a valley without a mobile phone signal. After we left the village, I had a call from an unknown number. It was Public Health England. The woman was very brusque and informed me that a routine swab taken at St Thomas' the week before had shown that H had a severe infection which required antibiotics and that anyone who had been in contact with her had to have an inoculation. Obviously, myself and the family we were with had to be treated. The children were not too keen on the jabs and H was really embarrassed. After returning home and speaking to the EB nurse she was very surprised at all the fuss, saying that some EB patients have infections and they rarely pass them on.

I was also lucky enough to have friends in lovely parts of the country and so we visited St Ives, Brighton, Nottingham and the Lake District. On one of our visits to St Ives when H was about three years old, she was sitting on the table in the kitchen where I had lanced a blister, when she slipped and damaged her face, hand and knee. I reacted in my usual way, mopping up the blood and dressing the wounds, but when I looked at my friends, I realised how upsetting it was for them. I had become hardened to accidents and it also made me realise how much H took it all in her stride.

As well as our holidays in the UK, we also went abroad, usually to see my brother in Spain but later on we ventured further afield.

Being in a hot country, fewer clothes were worn and when H was quite young there was the sympathetic "Ahh" from people, seeing a baby/toddler in dressings. But as she got older the "Ahhhs" changed to "Ugh". We spent a long time discussing it and decided that the only way to deal with it was to smile. The person/s would either smile back or look away. The ones who smiled back would sometimes ask what she had done, which gave the ideal opportunity to explain about EB.

On holiday in Spain H loved crazy golf and pool, usually with Uncle Dai. She tended to play crazy golf in the same way as pool and used the end of the club to push the golf ball through the holes. When playing pool, she used the cue one-handed pushing the ball. It was a great way to win. At the local bar one evening a little boy of about four came in, H, who was about eight, was playing pool, he stood staring at her for a long time, she smiled at him and he smiled back. The parents looked very uncomfortable, then he said in a broad northern accent: "Is she poorly?" (pronounced purely). H explained she had a skin condition, and had to be very careful not to bang herself, keeping it very simple. They then had a game of pool, but every person who came into the pub, he would stop and say: "Be careful, she's poorly", and then carry on with the game. We saw him several times on holiday and he acted like her bodyguard. His parents were lovely and asked all sorts of questions about EB. Children are often far more accepting of differences than adults. What happens?

On another occasion in Spain, we were walking along the front on a Sunday evening. Dai was pushing the wheelchair and I was behind chatting to Dai's partner. Two elderly Spanish women pointed at H and made a comment about the sun. My brother, who spoke Spanish replied to them in Spanish. They tutted and hurriedly walked on. I asked him what he had said and apparently, he told them that it wasn't sunburn, and when H was cured, they would still be ugly! My brother was very protective. The strange thing was that H was wearing trousers and the only damaged skin were her hands and elbows. It's unusual to get sunburn on your elbows.

In another of his protective days, Dai appeared at the swimming pool in the apartment where they lived. We were sitting under the umbrella after both having a swim. I was surprised to see him as he was usually at work all day and we only saw him in the evening. He looked around the pool, had a quick swim and disappeared. I questioned him later in the evening, and, apparently a little German man staying at the apartment block had complained about H being in the pool as they thought she was contagious and they could catch something.

As Dai and his partner were residents in the block, they knew the receptionist very well and so she told Dai rather than me, she was disgusted and devasted, she knew about H's condition but was unable to explain it to the man. As Dai couldn't find him, he left a message with the receptionist to tell the man that a big Englishman was looking for him. I carried leaflets in various languages given to me by DEBRA explaining about EB and that it wasn't contagious, which was a less aggressive way of explaining. We never saw him, and the receptionist kept the leaflet and I gave her others in different languages, just in case.

One evening, H and I were returning to the apartment leaving Dai at another bar. We called in on our way home to a friend's bar to have a nightcap. I had a Cointreau with ice. H had a Guinness. One became two quite large drinks. By the time we left the bar to walk along the promenade, both of us were feeling the effects. There is no rail between the prom and the beach and a drop of several feet. I managed with H's directions to keep to the prom and was more than delighted when we reached the apartment. I did wonder if you can be booked for being drunk in charge of a wheelchair.

Dai always collected coins for H (shrapnel as Dai referred to it). The collection was in a very large whiskey bottle. Each evening I would empty some of the coins from the bottle so that H could count them, put them in her purse and exchange them at Dai's local bar, where they were grateful for change and kind enough to give her larger denominations of coins or notes. On this particular occasion, we were late leaving the apartment as dressings had taken longer than usual. Dai was waiting at the bar and his partner had gone ahead to meet him.

As we were leaving the apartment, H realised that she had forgotten her money and so I tipped some out in her lap and told her to count them on the way to the bar. As we were crossing the road on the zebra crossing at the bottom of the hill, a couple coming towards us threw money into her lap. I immediately stopped and tried to explain but the couple smiled and walked on and we were left in the middle of the road with very cross motorists tooting their horns. I was embarrassed and upset that anyone would think we were begging and recounted the tale to Dai. I was amazed that instead of the same reaction as me, he laughed and said: "What a brilliant way to get beer money!" All H did was laugh – I was fighting a losing battle there.

As H got older, she loved having holidays with friends in different parts of the country, by then Carly, Nik and Claire were experts in bandaging and so I had no worries about them going away. Apart from when they went to Weymouth to the caravan and decided to take H on to the stony beach, I've no idea exactly what happened, but they didn't do it again. What happens on holiday, stays on holiday. At one point H and I were lucky enough to go to the flat belonging to the Spanish DEBRA. A beautiful three-bedroomed flat in Marbella. We walked up to meet the staff who were based above their DEBRA charity shop, it was only a small organisation, but they were lovely people who made us very welcome. With that in mind, H, Carly and Claire went for a week and had a brilliant time. The swimming pool was on the roof and Claire and Carly used it, but because H's back was so open, the water dragged the dressings down, making it too painful, she didn't venture into the water. However, Claire and Carly were not going to be beaten, they bought a large rubber ring, covered it with a towel to prevent rubbing, and lifted H until she was sitting in it. The only part that got wet was her bottom and her feet. I have a lovely photo with H in a swimsuit, t-shirt and hat lounging in the ring. Clever girls. Of course, they then had to go to Euro Disney, Nik, Carly and H had a weekend there. It was many years since I had taken her when she was about six, but her love of Disney had not diminished, in fact, the three of them were

Disney-mad. Armed with Disney headbands I took them to St Pancras and when I collected them, they were exhausted and voiceless, but so happy.

We had a holiday in Cyprus which was very interesting. We were sitting in the lobby one afternoon and H was in her wheelchair, I was sitting on a settee with my feet resting on her footrests. There was a sudden movement and a lady fell down the stairs. H accused me of pushing the wheelchair but it appears there was a tremor, according to the staff it was four on the Richter Scale and only lasted a few seconds. They were so blasé about it, and I guess they were used to it, but it certainly made me think how vulnerable they are.

We also visited Lanzarote with Jackie and all had henna tattoos, nearly as good as a tattoo, but not quite. When we went to Venice we travelled from Heathrow, and playing spot the celebrity, saw Philip Schofield who gave us a lovely wave, and Julie Walters and her daughter in the toilets who agreed to give us an autograph, a great way to start a holiday.

H always liked adventures, and so when Jackie and Rich, Jackie and Rob planned a holiday, it was to go to Toronto, Canada. Niagara Falls and the CN Tower were on the list. Sadly, Jackie and Rob couldn't go and so just the four of us went. Niagara Falls was amazing although H didn't agree. Boats were never her thing and I'd forgotten it. She went greener and greener, even as we got wetter, saying: "Wet, wet, wet" didn't make her smile. I should have remembered from boat trips over to France, and when, in my wisdom, I thought the hovercraft to Guernsey would be a good idea as it was much quicker, all that happened was that H was sick at a more rapid pace. The boat trip at Niagara Falls was not a great success for her, but the next day we went to the CN Tower. Direct drops are not my thing, I'm OK looking out from a height, up a mountain, but not from tall buildings, looking directly down.

Worse still the CN Tower has a glass floor. I closed my eyes as I pushed her in the chair onto the glass floor, she decided to get out, and she and Rich lay on the glass floor looking down. Jackie and I took photos and then Jackie took one of me which was blurred as my legs were shaking so much. It was an amazing holiday.

When we got home H booked us into a hotel in Blackpool to see the lights in November, just so that she could go up the tower. It was just her and I, and so I had to push the chair over the glass floor, luckily it is only a small square and so I was able to keep my feet on the carpet on either side of the glass and look ahead. I was fine until the man in charge said: "I don't know why you're doing that, there's glass under the carpet". Thanks, mate!

Another adventure was with Jackie (AJ as she became known by H: Aunt Jac). Sadly, Rob died the same year as Dad and so Jackie came with us on holiday. H always wanted to go to Disney, in Florida. We went for two weeks of the summer holidays, as we were both teachers. The hotel we stayed in was lovely, and we set off on our first day with great excitement. We went early as it was very hot during the day. We saw the parade, went on rides, and had a lovely time. We were heading back to the hotel and the heavens opened, we got so wet and H got even wetter sitting in the chair, with a big puddle in her lap. The taxi driver wasn't fazed by it and we dripped into the cab and out again. We got back to the hotel and decided to get into the hot tub. There were only two people in there, who got out and so we warmed up. H kept her back out but warmed up the rest of her body.

After about ten minutes, a member of staff came and said there had been a complaint from another visitor because of H's skin. They were worried it was contagious, we assured him that it was not, and explained the condition. We stayed in for a few more minutes, then went to do H's dressings. Jackie had her own room and soon came and knocked at the door. She is a very calm person, usually, but boy was she livid. She had been down and complained to the manager about H's treatment, and they had apologised. She came back for leaflets not only in English but also in German, as the tourist was German (not again!). She took the leaflets back down and a few minutes later we had complimentary hot chocolate, cookies and sweets from the hotel. No wine!

The next day the staff were so nice to us, as we set off even earlier to the park with the idea of leaving the park before the threatened thunderstorm. Like something out of the three pigs' story, unfortunately, it came earlier and so we still got wet, but this time H wouldn't go in the hot tub. The next part of our holiday was at Pete's Beach which again was lovely, and they had a big wheelchair which could be taken on the beach. It looked like it was made from giant Meccano. The only problem was that Jackie and I could push it straight, but it took considerable strength to turn it around and so for a while we ended up pulling it backwards until we could work it out. It was either that or leaving H on the beach.

Flo came over from Canada one year, so we decided that our holiday the following year would be with Flo on Prince Edward Island (PEI). It was a beautiful Island and we had a great time finding out about the Inuit people. It was the first time we had decided to take up our pharmacy's offer of getting our feeds from the local pharmacy on PEI, since our pharmacy could liaise with the one on PEI. They also offered me the facility for dressings to be organised, but I decided we would just start with the feeds. Good job I didn't agree to them preparing dressings since the feeds were three days late in getting to the pharmacy on PEI. Luckily, I had taken two bottles with me and we made up for the lack of feeds by giving her all her favourite foods: tuna pasta bake, pancakes and of course chocolate orange.

Nearer to home, H went camping with Lorraine and Pete. She enjoyed it but I think doing the dressings was always a challenge for them, however, they coped.

Travel was always part of our fun.

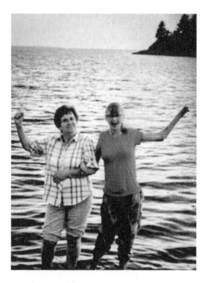

Aunty Flo Jo and H in Canada.

# 6

# Secondary school and other activities- (2001-2006)

My choice of secondary school was different from H's. She wanted to go with her friends, the local authority wanted her to go to the one with a physically impaired unit (catchy title). We went to look around both schools. The authority one rang alarm bells when they said that there were plenty of TAs who could take care of her needs. The problem was that the young boy with EB who had visited H in hospital didn't have very severe EB and required very little support, he went to this school, and they obviously thought EB was the same for every sufferer. H was horrified that anyone from a group of fifteen TAs could pierce blisters and dress wounds. I too was concerned about the training. All people mean well but sometimes a little knowledge is a dangerous thing.

We held a meeting at the school, where H wanted to go, with the Head Teacher, SENDCO and the wonderful Mary and it was decided that providing Lorraine was willing to transfer with her, then she could attend the school. We also discussed the need for other TAs to become trained as backups, just as they were in her two previous schools. There were two medical rooms, so one was able to be used for H with very few adaptions.

I can't say that the school was brilliant academically, but the staff were wonderful and very flexible in adapting the curriculum where they could. I still have the lamp she made in metalwork, I suspect with quite a lot of support from the teacher and Lorraine, it's beautiful in the garden in the summer; and a silk butterfly print she made in art, again with support from her teacher and Lorraine, this hangs in the hall.

Although H still went swimming, it soon became apparent that it was beginning to hurt her back. The downside of having the gastrostomy was that she had to sleep on her back, this seemed to cause friction which meant her back was continuously an open wound. Sadly, her back never healed and H rarely went swimming again.

In secondary at that time, it was quite difficult to adapt the PE, so it's good that things have changed. I became aware that H was spending a lot of time in her wheelchair, especially for quick movement around the school, which had never been an issue in the primary school, as generally they were in the same class and she was able to get up and move around the class. She showed a real interest in drama, being very dramatic all her life! And so, besides the drama lessons at school, she also joined a drama group on a Saturday morning. It was an amazing group of people, she did acting, singing (a voice like her mother – ummm!) and even dancing. Box ticked, fun, movement and building up leg muscles.

School was still a social event for H. As one of her reports read 'Heather will talk to anyone, at any time, about anything'. She had a small group of friends, went for sleepovers to those children whose parents had confidence in dealing with any issues which may occur; and we had many sleepovers with one, two or many more friends.

She also had a couple of great teachers who included her in their skiing trips in Austria. Although she was unable to ski, it was organised for her to have a sledge and an instructor. Lorraine went with her, but that didn't stop me from being concerned, but no need, she had a great time, so much so, that she went the following year.

H loved adventures and so I took her in a balloon, along with Mum/Nana. We left early in the morning from Littlecote House and landed in Newbury. It was a wonderful experience but slightly embarrassing when I asked about flying back, forgetting that it's the wind that makes the balloon travel and unless it changed directions, the only way of getting back was by Land Rover. Getting H out of the basket was easier than I thought, but getting Mum out proved to be challenging, her Parkinson's was quite advanced by then.

The following year we went on a helicopter ride with Aunt Jac, and then for her birthday, she had a glider lesson. But I drew the line at a parachute jump, luckily, they wouldn't insure her.

At secondary school some of the children struggled with understanding H's condition, even the ones who had been in primary school with her. One particular boy saw it as a perk that H left the class early to avoid mass movement but failed to realise that she was always first in the next lesson. In fact, he actually said, I wish I had an electric wheelchair to zoom around in and not have to walk – really!

Another girl started to make uncomplimentary remarks

about H. Typical teacher, I asked what she had done to her. H replied that if I was an ordinary mum, I would defend her, this made me realise that I needed to differentiate between mum and teacher. A restorative justice session was set up, which I think was successful in that both girls steered clear of each other and hardly ever spoke again.

Dressings every day, six monthly hospital visits continued to both hospitals, organised so that we saw a consultant once every three months, either at our local hospital or GOSH. Three-monthly eye appointments at our local hospital and eye check-ups at GOSH. My dentist took on H's care but consulted with the GOSH dentist. That was our life and it became the norm, as any RDEB family will know. Eventually, you get used to fitting things in as well as trying to enjoy the fun things of life. They become part of your routine, just like eating and cleaning your teeth.

During secondary school, a friend asked H to become godmother to the little boy she was adopting. She was delighted and he became her little prince. He was deaf and she made a real effort to learn how to sign, as I did but with less success. They became firm friends, even more so when she could drive and they would go for a Costa at regular intervals. My friend went on to adopt two more girls, who also became close to H. One had brittle bones, who she referred to as "Gob on Wheels" (in the nicest possible way) and the other was her partner in crime. I think mostly because it was criminal the amount of mess they made when baking cakes in my kitchen.

H constantly wanted her ears pierced, I held out for so long, and then eventually gave in. We found a very nice lady who read all the EB literature I gave her and then gave me instructions for the care afterwards. It went well, without any problems, but I guess we were over-cautious and over the top with the medical care. H loved having pierced ears and wore her earrings every day, and enjoyed having new ones for birthdays and Christmas.

Ant Jac had an interest in dolls' houses and bought H a room box which H made into a sweet shop, and then she was hooked, she added another box to the top and made a flat and above that a roof garden. The second house we got was three stories with staircases. The ground floor was an old-fashioned pub called "The Skerry Arms", which was my project. The second floor was an Italian restaurant, of course. This was H's project and had jugs of sangria and plates of spaghetti bolognese, which were made by another friend who was also into the miniature world. The top floor was an office, with the latest computers and a laptop. The final house was a hairdresser/beautician, all in black and white and called "A Cut Above The Rest". There were so many tiny things: hair rollers, hair dryers, nail varnish - she had great fun doing it.

We were running out of space to display the houses when she changed her hobby interest to jewellery-making. H started to make earrings, bracelets, and necklaces for everyone. I was amazed at how well she coped, as by this time her hands were becoming more restricted. She never wanted hand surgery, and I never tried to force her to have it, as she always seemed to find a way around obstacles. I'm guessing her small fingers were quite useful in making jewellery.

She used to refer to her hands and arms as her T-Rex arms, but only she was allowed to say it about herself. Later, she even made sixty wine glass decorations to go around the base of the glass. These were for Lorraine's daughter's wedding and were bands with beads the colour of the bridesmaids' dresses with a heart saying: "Thank you", which people could have to take home as a memento of the day. I thought she had taken on too much, especially when her hand started to bleed as she was using the pliers, but she was determined and over a period of time, she achieved the task.

H finished secondary school when she was sixteen. Her school results weren't brilliant. She did well in English, but Maths eluded her, just like her mother, and it took three attempts to achieve the standard she wanted. She did brilliantly in RE (Religious Education) and IT (Information Technology). From the time she was in Year Eight onwards, the school was in constant turmoil, with head teachers changing regularly and so many of the children were let down by the system at that time.

The school went on to become an Academy which included my school, and for me this became challenging, but this story is about H and so enough to say that professionally, the next few years were interesting. H left school in the summer of 2006, and like most of her year group, went to the prom. Dressed in a beautiful pink, yes pink, dress, she looked lovely and I was so proud of her. They had a stretch limo and not only did the family come to see them, but friends and neighbours, making them feel like celebrities. She still looked so young compared to the other girls but was gaining confidence.

Two women living together in a house during menstruation can be challenging, but gradually we became used to each other's mood swings, however, my menopause was a different thing. I got so cross with H at one point that I packed her bags and took her to Lorraine's house. Identifying flash point times was quite a skill, but we eventually knew when to avoid each other.

During H's time at secondary school and beyond we became more adventurous in our holidays, less reliant on others, and more able to travel by ourselves. For one of my special birthdays, we went to Venice. Pushing a wheelchair, pulling a case, bags on the handlebars of the wheelchair, and boxes with feeds loaded onto H's lap, became the norm and we had it down to a fine art. At the airport, people were always helpful and usually, the staff on the plane were as well. We were flying with British Airways and I was expecting good service.

The first incident was when they refused to put the chair in the hold at the gate, and said we had to use an airport one, putting mine in the luggage hold straight away. Having travelled many times to Spain with a variety of companies, I knew they could take the chair from us at the gate, so we stood our ground and they backed down. After going through security, which was always a challenge, we got into duty-free. H informed me that the reason she didn't want an airport wheelchair was that we would have had to have a porter to push it (health and safety), and that meant that she couldn't spend as much time in duty-free testing all the perfumes.

The plane trip was uneventful until we were just about to land, it was rather bumpy and H decided to be sick. Luckily, she held on until I found a bag. As we left the plane, seat padding over my arm, handbag over my shoulder, medical bag on my arm, guiding H and carrying the sick bag in my hand, we got to the front of the plane and I ask if one of the crew could take the sick bag and put it in the bin. She pointed to the bin on the other side of the plane, and I had to leave H to put it in the bin. I was not best pleased. We got through customs and found our water taxi waiting.

Arriving at the hotel I looked for my reading glasses to pay the taxi driver and realised that at that moment my reading glasses had also been in my hand and they were now in the bin on the plane.

~

H spent a very happy holiday, reading the menus and sorting out the money. Venice was a lovely place to visit, but at that time not very wheelchair friendly. I hadn't realised that the bridges had steps, I thought they were like the one in the *Three Billy Goats Gruff*, a smooth run. I spent the whole holiday saying get out, hold onto the rail and walk up the steps, bump the wheelchair up the steps, get back in and bump H and the chair down the other side. Despite all this and low-flying pigeons, we had a wonderful holiday.

Italy became a favourite destination for us, and we went to the Lakes region, enjoyed the weather, the food and the lovely company of people staying at the hotel. We walked miles, at least I did, and being on the flat it was easy to push the chair, but I think watching H consume large quantities of Italian ice cream was magical. In fact, she ate so much one day that she didn't need her pump. Who knew such things could give so much pleasure?

For H's fifteenth birthday, a group of our friends went with us to New York. The reveal of the upcoming holiday was at our favourite Italian restaurant, Rob had bought it as a surprise for Jackie, Rich for the other Jackie and me for H. All were presented with an apple and a photo of New York, the Jackies both guessed but H was completely flummoxed. Eventually, she got it and was so excited.

The journey there was great but the entry to New York was challenging. Going through security and being asked for fingerprints proved interesting. Due to constant trauma, H did not have fingerprints, the passport official asked if she had amputations, to which she showed him all her limbs. I explained the condition and he tried to find it on his system, when he couldn't find anything, he referred us to Police Security. I could only describe the room as being like something out of *Hill Street Blues* (for those old enough to remember), there were three police officers behind a high desk, who all leaned across the desk and asked H what she had done. Needless to say, she burst into tears.

In the corner of the room, there was a glass booth, out of this came another officer, obviously in charge. He beckoned us into the booth and I sat down, we both explained the situation and I gave him a leaflet. He was very apologetic and kind and wished us a happy holiday, assuring me that the condition would be added to the system. As we left his office, the other police officers had come from behind the desk and made a guard of honour, smiling and wishing us "a nice day".

We re-joined our group outside by the carousel, only to be met by a very large lady security guard holding the feeds' box above her head saying: "Who does this belong to?" My caring friends all pointed to me. H had by this time regained her composure, and when we approached the security guard and explained what it was, she looked blankly at us. So, H pulled up her top and pointed to the gastrostomy button. The confusion was then in the eyes of the security guard, she didn't actually apologise, but pointed out that she thought it was bird feed. As we wanted to get on with our holiday, although I was tempted, I never said that if it was bird feed it would have said so.

We travelled into New York City in a stretch limo, the hotel was lovely. We saw all the usual sights including being fast-tracked up to the top of the Empire State Building, "cripple perks" as H said. AJ was appalled by this but as H said, I can say it but you can't! H and I took a trip on the Ferris wheel inside the Toys 'R' Us store. It had to be done. Everyone was so kind, especially the mounted police who took time to have photos taken with H.

Our next holiday with our friends was in Rome. Crossing to the Colosseum, Rob decided he would take over pushing the wheelchair across the cobbles to help me out. He nearly got H run over as he was looking in the wrong direction as he crossed.

This was pretty much the same as when I took H to Paris and tried to cross the Champs-Elysees. Besides the crossing being on a countdown, and therefore having to stop in the middle of the dual carriageway, there wasn't enough space in the centre of the road for both me and H in the wheelchair, so I decided my bottom was more important than her footrests. Luckily nobody ran her over.

Our trip to Rome was cut short and we had to return early as my dad was in hospital and not expected to live. We arrived at the hospital, to find him sitting up in bed saying: "Hello my darlings what are you doing here?" The consultant was very apologetic and Dad survived for another year.

As we missed out on our Rome trip, we decided to go to southern Ireland in the summer. I hired a car at the airport, which was just large enough to get our luggage in. The trip was great. We saw elephants on roundabouts (a local circus nearby), visited the Waterford Crystal Factory and generally met lovely people and saw beautiful scenery. The only downside was that H was too young to sample the Guinness.

H was also lucky enough to have people who wanted her as a bridesmaid. It was always a bit of a challenge to make sure she was wearing the same as the other bridesmaids, but the flexibility to cover her arms and neck if necessary helped.

The first time she was a bridesmaid, she was only six and she was asked by a woman who had a child in my class at school. The girls (four in all) were wearing Bo Peep-type dresses and carrying hoops, all in different colours. To say that the other girls were much larger than H would be an understatement. It was the hottest day of the year, and I was in charge of dressing the girls and getting them to the church.

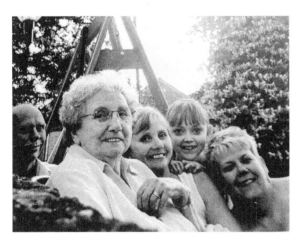

Lorraine, Pete, Mum, H and I in the garden.

H was easy compared to the others; I used a whole container of talcum powder to get them into their dresses. But it was a lovely day. The next one was when she was a flower girl for Aunt Jac and Rob. She had a lovely blue dress in the same fabric as Jackie's and was instructed to take Jackie's bouquet and hold it for the service. We didn't realise there would be a table in front of them, and so when Jackie put the bouquet on the table, a little hand whipped around and took the bouquet off the table. She was doing what she was told.

My lovely friend Sal was the next and she and Doug got

married in beautiful Cornwall. The five girls were all of a similar age and wore sunflower dresses. It was a beautiful wedding, and the reception was at a friend's hotel with a pool. It was still at a time when H was able to go in the water without too much pain. The bridesmaids spent the whole afternoon playing in the water and then the very kind friends of Sal and Doug found me a room where I could do her dressings before we set off for home.

The last two were when she was older, and both were connected to Lorraine. On both occasions, the dresses were quite strappy at the top, but she was able to wear boleros to cover her arms and neck without looking out of place. The brides were both so accommodating. Being a bridesmaid was so exciting for her and people are so kind.

# 7

# College, car, and eye issues
# (2006-2010)

H decided to transfer to the local college to do 'A' levels and retake her dreaded Maths class. In those days the statement ceased at sixteen and so we were left wondering about medical support. Although there was a part-time first aider, it soon became evident that this wasn't enough. Education decided they weren't paying for a carer, social services decided they weren't paying either.

Then along came the social support advisor from DEBRA, armed with a pile of documents explaining why they might be breaking the law if the necessary adaptions were not made available. The authorities soon backed down and shared the cost, asking for Lorraine to transfer to the college with H. This meant that Lorraine had been with H from the age of three, all the way through her school and college years.

She loved college and met one of her best friends there. At first, she studied IT, Sociology, Photography and the dreaded Maths. She also liked the freedom it gave her to sit with her friends and chat.

H always had jobs to do in the house, but with her restrictions, it was important to find equipment to support her; a lightweight hoover, tin and lid openers, and an onion slicer. There was no excuse for her not helping with the housework and the cooking.

H turned sixteen in June before she went to college and was keen to start learning to drive, able to do so because of her disability. We tried her in my parents' car since both of them had given up driving, but the gears, handbrake and pedals were too much of a challenge. She decided to have a mobility car using some of her DLA (Disability Living Allowance). She selected an automatic pale blue Nissan Micra which was named "BeeBee", had a peg fitted on the wheel and an electric handbrake.

My parents, H and I took the car to the Lake District to see our friends, at this time she couldn't drive on the motorway, so I did, and she drove the scenic lanes. While we were there, I was reversing into a space next to a raised flower bed, and because the peg on the wheel was so easy to turn, I ended up hitting it. The car was less than three months old and in for repairs. I admitted it was my fault, although I still think the flower bed jumped out.

My lovely neighbour who was a driving instructor agreed to take H out driving and he donated half the cost of the lessons to DEBRA. I took him to one side and told him to take his time in getting her ready for her test. Less than four months later he said that she had to put in for a test as she was ready and a very good driver. Her test was on January 1st and she passed - at just sixteen and a half.

The first thing she did was to take fish and chips over to Nan and Grandad, and then take them for a drive in the car. I am always so grateful for that, as sadly my dad died the following month, and he saw her achieve driving in her car.

There was no stopping her then, she drove everywhere. When she didn't have lessons at college, she would drive with Sabrina over to see Mum, pop into town to do some shopping or go off to the cinema. On one shopping expedition, we went into Next, one of her favourite shops, she selected her outfits, and because we were going to lots of shops which were quite a way apart, I pushed her in the wheelchair. At the till, H handed over the clothes and got out her debit card. The girl at the till looked at me and said: "Does she want a bag?", I turned to H and said: "Do you want a bag?", she responded with: "No thank you," to me, and so I said to the girl: "No thank you". The action went completely over the girl's head but we laughed about it for ages afterwards.

H even decided that she wanted to be the one to drive to GOSH in London for hospital appointments. The first time she drove there I was on edge, but once I realised that I could now look around at the sights it was fantastic. Journeys home were always interesting as there were signs saying how long it would take between junctions, H took this as a challenge rather than the time it should take! She loved driving and it made me rather redundant for a while. But she was happiest behind the wheel.

I then began to understand how inconsiderate some drivers are about disabled parking. I have challenged this over the years, when able-bodied people without blue badges have parked in disabled spaces, not necessarily ones we wanted to go in, and sometimes when I have been on my own. Generally, when challenged, people would apologise, quite often saying they hadn't realised they were parking in a disabled spot (the big disabled sign on the ground is usually a give-away), or that they were only going to be a few minutes, but they often moved their car. But there have been occasions when I've been asked what it's got to do with me or told to f\*\*\* off. H used to get cross with me and tell me to leave it, otherwise, in her words: "You'll get punched". Even now I find myself going to challenge people parking without blue badges in disabled spaces and in my head, I hear a voice saying: "Leave it, Mumsie, you'll get punched!"

At about the same time, our visits to GOSH stopped and we were transferred to St Thomas' Hospital. It was a scary time for both of us; for H because it was all new and for me because I was leaving the support of all the wonderful staff at GOSH. Luckily for us, on our first visit, we were given our link nurse, Jane. Everything seemed very grown-up. The clinic at that point was in the old part of the building and less than adequate. Since then, a new purpose-built clinic has been created. I felt even more redundant since suddenly H was the adult and everything was referred directly to her, and the professionals even asked if H wanted me included in the conversation. It was a good learning curve as I was forced to admit that H was grown-up and suddenly, she started making all the decisions.

When H had been driving for about six months, getting an eye infection was a blow. At first, it appeared the same as her usual problem, when the eye became red and sore. We had drops for these occasions, to deal with the infection. She used the drops but after a couple of days nothing seemed to be improving, so H made an emergency appointment with our Ophthalmologist Consultant at the local hospital. The consultant saw her on a regular basis between our visits to GOSH to see our consultant there.

Unfortunately, she had been called away on an emergency and we saw her Registrar. I should have been wary when he admitted that he had never treated or seen someone with EB. He gave her more drops and sent her home. After two days the eye still had not improved and so we returned to the local hospital and saw our consultant, who sent us immediately to Moorfield Eye Hospital, as we were no longer at GOSH, and this was then the centre of excellence for EB.

A friend drove us frantically up to Moorfield, having no idea where we were going, taking an overnight bag as I was told we may have to stay in. They dropped us off and I went into the clinic to see the EB eye consultant. He saw us but then directed us to the children's department as he only dealt with adults over eighteen. We saw a consultant there who said that he didn't deal with EB as the children always went to GOSH to see the expert there. I burst into tears and he took pity on me and phoned GOSH, spoke with our eye consultant, who told us to come back to GOSH. I phoned my friends and told them to go home, got a taxi to GOSH and saw the consultant immediately. Sadly, H had to have an operation which removed her cornea and lens. The cornea was replaced with a temporary one.

So, she was blind in one eye and had dodgy vision from constant scarring in the other. We were in the hospital for a week and I went home for a day by train to collect more clothes. Luckily I didn't need dressings as they were all available at GOSH.

Now H's body was at St Thomas's but her eyes were at GOSH! H always said that whoever gave their cornea, gave her back her life. This mix-up doesn't happen anymore as there is a gradual transfer from one hospital to the other between the ages of sixteen and eighteen. For the next eighteen months, we went to GOSH monthly to see our amazing consultant.

When the time came for the stitches to come out, he very kindly organised for us to go to his private clinic in Slough, which was much easier to get to. He offered H something to keep her calm, but as usual, she refused and I watched as he approached her eye with an instrument to cut the stitches. Apparently, I went a funny shade of green and was taken out and given some water; H just sailed through it.

We continued our visits to GOSH for the next 18 months, seeing our consultant and he then arranged for us to see a lady about contact lenses. She worked both at GOSH and Moorfield and became a wonderful support to us. After eighteen months, we saw our consultant at GOSH for the last time. The cornea had taken and it wouldn't be replaced until it was rejected, which it never did.

We had to leave GOSH, as the consultant told us H was too old to be there and wasn't insured! By this time, she was over eighteen. We transferred to the adult department at Moorfield and saw the man we had first seen when we went to Moorfield, along with our lovely contact lens lady. She tried all sorts of lenses until with the consultant's permission H's vision was good enough to be able to drive again. We continued going to Moorfield every six months and seeing our lovely lady, who tweaked the lens to give her good day driving vision, although she only drove short distances in the dark.

We found a great car park near to Moorfield which only cost us £8 for the day. The lady who ran it became a friend, she had a big dog called Tyson who would come to see H and was gentle with her. H always gave her £10 for the car parking, £8 for the fee and £2 for a treat for Tyson. I'm sure he knew her car and was waiting for us when we arrived.

H also had glasses to help her other eye and wonderful

glasses which she could put on at night when she took her contact lenses out. H already had big eyes, but these glasses made her look like an owl. Initially, I had to put her lenses in, but when it became apparent that I was useless at it, H did it, balancing the lens on her hand between her finger and thumb (she couldn't use just her finger as it was bent and slightly fused). She then balanced her elbow on her knee and lifted the knee, hand and lens to her eye. She was a complete contortionist. It was amazing to watch!

Eighteen months later and she was back to driving, but it had an impact on her education. I always felt really guilty that I hadn't acted quicker and maybe the infection wouldn't have been so catastrophic. But that's how it is for EB parents, who always feel guilty about something.

Getting back to driving gave her independence and this is when she developed her love of cars. Her first one, the pale blue Nissan Micra was lovely, but she wanted something different for her next car and after the Micra went back and she was able to drive again, she selected a dark blue Mitsubishi. This was followed three years later by a black Peugeot and then, as she loved this car, at last, another Peugeot in her favourite colour; orange. For her last car, she had done lots of research and selected a fast VW which she loved driving. I have that car now and I love driving it too.

At college, during the period of time that she had eye issues, she still managed to complete and pass all her subjects, doing the work, but with the help of a scribe. All except IT. She had completed the first year and was persuaded to attend the lectures in the second year but not take the exam, putting this off until the following year when she would be nineteen.

Unfortunately, the course was changed and so at eighteen, she had to start an IT course all over again. Alongside the IT course, she studied other subjects, but by the time she finished the courses, she was twenty and had had enough of college, although she had several GCSEs and 'A' levels. Her initial plan was to go to university at eighteen, but with eighteen months of eye issues and four years at the local college, it was enough. H decided she wanted a job. Lorraine stayed on as staff at the college and H looked for a job.

During her time at college, she turned eighteen and so we had a big party for her. Her friends, my friends, and our friends were all there. It coincided with our friends from Australia being over and Dai came from Spain. The only sad point was that neither Dad nor Rob was there as they had died the previous year. As always, H's birthday went on for at least a month, partying with her friends, meals with her family and day trips out. H always did birthdays and Christmases to an epic level.

It was during her time at college that her love of musicals and concerts developed. For the next ten years, she was all over the place seeing Olly Murs (ten times), Ed Sheeran, Pink, Panic at the Disco, George Ezra and others I can't remember. But I do remember going to see Michael Buble at the O2. Usually, disabled seats tend to be at a platform at the side or at the back, with not always the best views, but at the O2 we were virtually on the stage, and it was almost as though he was singing to us. H also took me to see David Essex in Cardiff, I was in my element until H pointed out that she was the youngest person in the audience by about thirty years.

Her love of musical theatre began when I took her to see *Chitty Chitty Bang Bang*. From then on, she was hooked, we went to *The Lion King*, *Wicked*, *War Horse*, *Evita* and many others. But she would never come with me to see *Phantom of the Opera* or *Les Miserables*, which she referred to as "Less Miserable". So those were the ones I went to with my friends.

She was so excellent at planning our trips that I rarely had anything to do except pack the dressings.

By this time dressings had changed so much since she was a baby. H obviously couldn't dress her back, but she did a great deal of the rest of her body herself. The regime was polymem on her back and Mepitel to hold it in place. The polymem absorbed much of the exudate which became quite heavy during the day and so the mepitel held it in place. We then used lyofoam which acted as padding and as sometimes it was difficult to source, I used to wash it. As it wasn't right next to her skin, I wasn't too worried about the non-bio washing liquid affecting her skin. However, the downside was that if I inadvertently put the net bag with the lyofoam in the washing machine with something with a strong colour, I could end up with rainbow-coloured lyofoam, which was always a laughing point in our dressing regime.

The whole dressing which was right down her back was held on by beige Tubifast. H had long since voiced her hatred of bandages. The rest of her dressings on arms, legs, hands or feet were either Mepilex, Transfer or ordinary Mepilex and a variety of Tubifast to hold in place – green, blue or yellow. I still had a small piece of red which I kept because that was the colour used on her leg and hand when she was born, and it was always a reminder of how tiny she was. I always washed the Tubifast, to try and save the NHS money and also because H preferred the texture and the smell after the Tubifast had been washed. We also ended up sewing the Tubifast so that they fitted, because, even though there were many colours for different sizes, occasionally some were either too tight or too loose, so taking them in made the Tubifast fit snuggly.

Initially, I did all the ordering of dressings, later on, we did it together, and then H took over this task. At first, I had to get them from the local pharmacy. Luckily, I had a car with a big boot, as there were usually about fifteen large boxes, including the feeds. The binmen always knew when I had collected the prescription as there were large cardboard boxes which I had to break down and put into the recycling boxes, which was quite a task.

The feed bottles were even more of a challenge as they would not be taken by the binmen without the silver heat-sealed tops being cut off. It was impossible to peel them off without breaking your nails or cutting your hands, so I used to slit open the top to pour the contents into the pump container. This left me with the challenge of cutting the tops off for recycling. I broke many knives trying to do this, but we did our bit for recycling.

Eventually, DEBRA was able to organise a company to deliver dressings, which made life simpler and then I only had to get all the medical delivery into the vast medical cupboard upstairs. As well as the dressings, there were medicines, eye drops and other random medical supplies. It was always a challenge to get it all in the cupboard. The local pharmacy still had to prescribe the feeds, as they came from a different money source. We also had a separate delivery of the gastrostomy equipment, as that came from the area health authority. We did eventually go back to our local pharmacy since they organised a delivery service and that meant we could have dressings and feeds delivered.

I was grateful when H took over the ordering, and although we still did a stock check together, she spoke to the people who dealt with the orders, and, if necessary, when stock wasn't delivered. She always loved a spreadsheet and so was in her element tracking everything.

H was given direct payments when she was sixteen, after a social worker became involved when H transferred to college. I suspect we could have had them before then, but if you don't know then you can't apply for them. It always seems amazing to me that no social worker checked on us after we left hospital when H was born. I didn't really want one, but it might have been useful to have one to navigate which benefits we could have accessed.

Initially, the direct payments were used for Lorraine to come and do dressings a couple of times a week which gave me respite. H always dealt with her direct payments and when friends began doing her dressings, I was grateful for this as it seemed very complicated with hours, holidays and tax. Carly and Nik's dressings sessions almost always turned into chatting sessions and makeup, hair and clothes sessions, so I'm not sure how long the dressings actually took, but they were often upstairs for many hours. By this time H was having showers rather than baths as those were too painful for her. Showers were quicker, as previously when she had baths, I could prepare and cook a Sunday roast while she was still in the bath. The direct payments were also used to allow her to go on holiday with her friends, and for me to go on holiday, when her friends would move into our house and do dressings etc. And I suspect – party!

I found that the most bizarre part of the medical dressing organisation was getting rid of the full sharps box containing the needles used to pierce blisters. At first it was easy, I would just take it to the doctors' surgery, but then it changed to become the responsibility of the local authority. They would only collect it on a certain day and time, which was when I was at work. When I pointed this out, they told me to leave it on the doorstep. In my eyes that was a bit dangerous! My lovely neighbour agreed to wait in for them. There wasn't really much flexibility from our local authority.

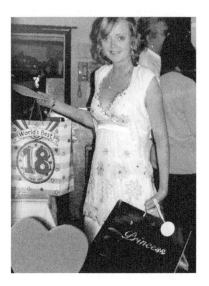

H's 18th birthday.

# 8

# Animals

H has always been a great lover of animals. When she was born, my parents had a dog called Tandy, who despite being blind, was very placid and allowed H to cuddle up to her and even put blankets over her. Sadly, Tandy died when H was two and despite my parents always having dogs, they decided that a dog, particularly a puppy, might damage H if the dog jumped up.

As time went by, I noticed that dogs in general seem to recognise that they needed to be gentle with H. Dai's dog, Cookie, in Spain, bounced around and jumped at everyone except H. He would nuzzle up to her, sit next to her and lay on her lap. Our next-door neighbour had a massive German shepherd dog called Scooby. He would ignore me, despite how much I tried to be friends with him, but would go straight to H and lean against her. Considering he was about seven stones in weight, I was always surprised that he didn't knock her over, although I suspect it was a gentle lean. Even so, a dog was out of the question, with me working etc.

For one of her birthdays, when H was still young, Jac

decided to buy her a rabbit. They went to buy it at the pet shop and came back with a tiny white rabbit called Binky Boo. Obviously, I did the cleaning out, because of the risk of H contracting an infection in her open wounds, but H was able to hold it on her lap with a cover over her legs and feed it with vast quantities of carrots and lettuce. She adored the rabbit but unfortunately, after she had had her for about two years, a fox broke into the hutch and took Binky. I didn't have the heart to tell H and so I said she had run away to join the other rabbits in the field. I kept this lie up until H was about sixteen.

H missed Binky and so we bought her a black and white rabbit. Initially, she wanted to call it Didcot, but there was no way that I was going to sound like a Station Master calling Didcot, so she decided to call him Patch. Patch was an indoor rabbit, well trained in using his litter tray, however, he did like wires and when I realised that I hadn't received any calls on the landline for over a week, I followed the telephone wire to find that he had chewed through it. Thank goodness it wasn't an electric cable. We were then very careful to lift or cover wires so that he couldn't get at them.

We also used to have the school rabbit at weekends, who was the size of a medium dog, despite when my class and I collected her, being told that she was a dwarf, she grew and grew. The class had named her Poppy when we thought she was going to be small. Some of the TAs were frightened of her, but she too was always gentle with H. Poppy was quite keen to get to Patch and vice versa, but we kept them apart. At weekends, and in the holidays, Poppy lived in the garden and wasn't bothered by foxes, I think they were scared of her. Patch lasted about three years and Poppy about five years.

At one of our trips to Marlborough Mop, Pete managed to win H two fish and bought her a pink fish tank with accessories. Needless to say, it was my responsibility to clean them out. Rob

(Jackie's husband) decided that the tank was too small and bought her a large one with a pump, so I made it his responsibility to clean it out when they came up once a week. The fish were called Maggie and Dennis, Pete and I helped name them, Maggie had a temper and was very much in control and Dennis had eyebrows. They were named after Maggie Thatcher and Dennis Healey. Pete and I thought it was funny. We had the fish for two years before Dennis died, which was probably quite good for fairground fish. So, Maggie swam around on her own.

Dai came down that summer and was out shopping with H, when he phoned me, and asked if I wanted fish. I thought he meant fish and chips for lunch, so I said yes. It turned out that he wanted to buy H another fish to replace Dennis. She rightly said that he needed to ask me. They came home with a replacement called Sherlock. The fish lived for another couple of years and then the tank went and I regained a large surface area in my lounge. They were fun while we had them.

I also used to hatch chicks or ducklings in the incubator at school. But they too had to come home at weekends, as they set off the alarms because of movement. The caretaker was OK about them during the week, but not so keen at weekends. H was always so gentle with them, and she particularly liked it when we hatched ducklings as after a few days they would swim in the bath or the paddling pool. H would give them lettuce and they would dive to get any that sank. Then she would gently dry them and put them back in the brooding pen.

H was a little confused the first time they ever came home as I put Smarties in their saucer containing feed, to attract their attention. She understood quickly, unlike one of the children in my classes who brought in ten tubes of Smarties to feed them. His mother was very embarrassed when she realised. It was an easy mistake to make!

The final triumph after years of saying no, was when I decided a cat would be alright if we got the right one. My dad was still worried about a cat scratching H, but Mum and I agreed that it was time, as H was about fourteen by this time. Luckily, I had a good friend with a cattery and she found the perfect cat.

Leah had been owned by a man, then his girlfriend moved in with two large male cats and they made Leah's life hell. The owner decided that Leah needed a good home, personally, I'd have got rid of the girlfriend! Leah was very nervous, and when I took H to see her without telling her my thoughts, I was rather worried that the cat was too nervous. H fell in love with her and when I said we could have her, H was so excited. The understanding was that we would give Leah a week to settle, and if she didn't, then my friend would take her back and try and find another home for her. Leah was a tiny black and white cat of four years old when we got her and died when she was twenty-one.

During the first week of having her, she spent all her time behind the microwave in the kitchen, which was at an angle in the corner. She came out at night and ate food, drank water and used her litter tray. Other than that, we didn't see her. I was just considering that I may have to return her to the cattery when one evening we were in the lounge watching television and she wandered into the lounge, jumped onto the settee and jumped up onto the back of the settee behind H. She settled herself down and that became her place.

As time went by, she would occasionally sit on a lap with a cover over the knees, but she preferred to be higher. I'm guessing that's what she did in her previous home to get away from the other cats. She ventured upstairs and would get under the covers in bed with H. But she always woke me in the morning to be fed, she was so light that I wouldn't hear her coming and when I opened my eyes, she would be staring at me. That could be scary first thing in the morning.

Leah also developed a liking for drinking fresh water from the bathroom tap and would sit and wait for it to be turned on. My neighbour who didn't particularly like cats, came in to feed her one day, while we were at the hospital, and said watching her drink from the tap made her smile so much that she had to stroke Leah. Leah also liked water from a glass, usually H's! So, we had to get her a glass just for her which was always left in the same place. That's not to say that sometimes she wouldn't go to somebody else's glass and dribble in that. Yuk! Leah was a particularly purry cat, in fact H referred to her as a "'appy cat", often having to turn the sound on the television up to drown the noise.

Leah was the light of her life, I'm sure she shared any problems with her. It took a long time for Leah to venture out, and when she did it was into the garden, where she would lie in the sun and become quite sweaty and rather smelly. She didn't mind being bathed or having her nails cut, which I did frequently to stop any chance of severe scratching. Sometimes at night Leah would try and get out of my bedroom window onto the flat roof. I was worried because of the local foxes, and although people said she would easily get away or avoid them, I still had in my mind what happened to Binky, and Leah was so small.

She was easy to get back inside by shaking her treat box, that was until she got older and could no longer hear, and on one occasion she went out the window and couldn't hear the treats being shaken, so I ended up climbing out after her to catch her with H cheering me on. From then on, the window was tied closed with a small gap, that even she couldn't get out of.

Probably the best adventures Leah had were when we

found out that she would happily sit on the back seat of the car with H, rather than in her carrier, where she would howl. H bought her a harness and she sat on a cover on H's knee, with the harness attached to the seat belt. She would go on journeys with us including to the care home where my mum eventually went for the last two years of her life. Occasionally we would also take Leah on the harness out for a short walk, although this wasn't quite as successful. With Leah's deafness came a change in her cry and purr, but she was still the same. I was Leah's servant but H was her person and the love of her life.

There were odd occasions when she got in the way and H had to avoid tripping over her. On one occasion Leah wanted feeding and walked in front of H, she fell over her and landed on the laminate floor, damaging her face and hands. There was blood everywhere, but all H could say was: "Feed Leah and then deal with me". When H told the story, she referred to face-planting the floor, but it could have been worse, as she'd only just put down her phone and that could have been damaged!

Christmas 2018, Leah began to lose weight and was very wobbly on her legs. Despite this, Leah still managed to play with all the toys H had bought her for Christmas and eat the treats. After Christmas, we took her to the vet. The veterinary nurse was someone H had gone to school with and she and the vet managed to keep Leah going until the end of January, and then we both agreed the time was right, we didn't want her in any more pain. We took Leah to the vet and H held her until she died. Leah gave us seventeen years of joy and love.

H's love of elephants started when we took a trip to South Africa. Obviously, she had her encounter with an elephant when it stole her ice cream, but this didn't seem to put her off.

The trip started with the usual preventative injections and our EB nurses gave me advice on these. It was suggested that H shouldn't have live vaccines and so that is why South Africa was selected as our destination. We had a two-centred holiday planned. In the first place we had a morning and evening trip to Kruger National Park, with our own guide, kindly organised to make sure H had plenty of room and wasn't at risk of being knocked. The safari was wonderful, seeing the "Big 5" but also a pack of wild dogs, which neither H nor I got excited about, but apparently was a very rare sight and lots of people got very animated.

We had an elephant experience with the local guide and got up close and personal; they are such wonderful large animals. The highlight of the first part of the trip was watching a crocodile on the lawn and a hippo in the water close by, followed by a man sitting with his gun. I had a swim in the pool, H didn't because of her back, and it was fascinating to watch the monkeys in the trees. I innocently asked where they had come from and the waiter said Kruger, then I stupidly said that I thought there was a fence surrounding Kruger and so how did they escape? H looked at me in disbelief and said, they swing and climb over the fence. Duhhh!

The second centre was a private game reserve, and from the time when I had booked, the accommodation had changed from chalet-style bungalows to ones in the heart of the reserve which looked like something out of the *Flintstones*. Not only did it have an inside shower but also an outside one, I used it once, but the noises of the animals were very loud, although I suspect it was because the noises were echoing. H said she'd shower in the indoor one.

On the first night we went to the restaurant which overlooked the reserve, which was full of beautiful views and lovely people. We had an evening safari, during which time the

Land Rover we were in hit a rut and broke its axle. While we were waiting for a replacement, the driver said it was safe to get out and wander around, although he did have a gun. The replacement Land Rover arrived and we all piled in. A minute later we turned a corner to find a lioness and cubs lying in the road. Very safe.

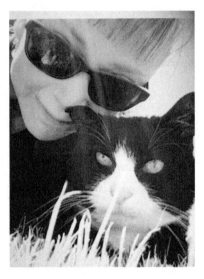

H and Leah - her 'little lady'.

The next day we had another elephant experience, but this time, it was very close up. The elephant was called Tambo, and the man in charge made him lie down so that he could explain all about the elephant. He selected H to keep Tambo quiet by feeding him a selection of food, including peanuts. At one point she stopped feeding Tambo, while she listened to the commentary, Tambo wasn't impressed and blew in her face. Despite this, she fell in love with the elephant, and couldn't wait to stand in front of Tambo and have her photo taken. She backed up until she was pressed against his knee so that he knew she was there. He was about three times her height and a gentle giant, although I wouldn't want to make him cross.

On the way back to the "hotel", there was a huge thunderstorm, which flooded the paths. I phoned reception and asked if dinner could be sent to our room as there was no way I could push the wheelchair to the reception and it was far too slippery for H to even attempt to walk. The lady in reception said she would get back to me, five minutes later, four men arrived at the door and carried the wheelchair with H to the restaurant, like she was some kind of princess. They didn't want us to miss dinner in the restaurant as there was entertainment as well. They were such kind people. It was a wonderful holiday and adventure and began H's love affair with elephants.

9

## H's calendar

H lived her life through her calendar. In the respect that she loved celebrations.

New Year's Eve was always spent with friends, sometimes we were together and sometimes she was just with her own friends. She always made a big fuss of my dad and celebrated his birthday, and even after he died, we went out for dinner and raised a glass to him. H loved giving, and Mothering Sunday was always special. We would go for a meal out the week before, as it was usually so crowded on the day, then lots of very personal presents on the day and often a drive out and a picnic in the car if it was cold. There was always a bouquet of flowers with freesias, my favourite flower.

Mum/Nana never got left out, with presents from both of us and H also used her pocket money to buy presents. Easter involved an Easter egg hunt with friends. June was Mum and H's birthday and so there was a three-to-four-week celebration. Presents and dinner with Mum, then with her friends and then a party, and there was always a cake. We often had a get-together in the garden with Pimm's and strawberries. July and

August were always summer holidays, if we were in Spain, it was sangria and paella. July was my birthday and I was always spoilt by H. October saw us going to Marlborough Mop to go on the big wheel, possibly with H going on the small rides with her legs under her chin, if the children came with us, followed by chips and a cheeseburger for me. On Firework Night, we had mulled wine, jacket potatoes and marshmallows, although they weren't my strong point as I tended to melt them.

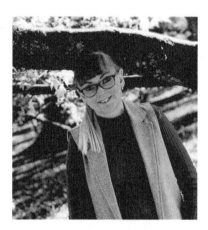

H in the autumn on her annual visit to Westonbirt Arboretum with Carly.

Carly and H loved to go to Westonbirt Arboretum to see the autumn leaves. Then it was preparation time for Christmas, with spreadsheets and lists. H loved giving and always planned very carefully what everyone would have. She organised for us to go to Christmas markets: the ones in Bath and Gloucester were always favourites; Christmas lights at Blenheim or Longleat; pantomimes, often in Swindon, Bristol or Oxford, but we did go to London one year which was amazing. We were usually in London in December for clinic and so we always took a walk along the South Bank and then drove around to see the lights. Christmas Day was taken up with presents, then lunch. Initially, I would cook for my parents, Jackie, Rob and her parents. Later on, we would go out for Christmas lunch, then afterwards, go back home on our own and wear Christmas pjs which H bought every year, and watch *Elf* and *Love Actually* on TV. Boxing Day we spent with Lorraine and Pete. H was a lover of Christmas.

# 10

# Work - (2020)

After four years at college, achieving her 'A' levels and GCSEs, despite having to start her IT 'A' level all over again due to her eye problems, H had exhausted her interest in full-time education. Although she could have stayed at home, lived on benefits and attempted some voluntary work, she was determined to get a job, so that she had, as she put it, her own money, not from the Government.

It was an interesting experience going to the Job Centre. To begin with, I had to go with her as there was no disabled parking space nearby and it was too far to walk. So, I pushed her in her manual chair. The first question after the preliminaries, was: "Is there any type of work you cannot do?" I refrained from saying anything, although I really wanted to say: "Probably not road laying". After a further discussion about H's condition: "No it's not eczema or psoriasis, you can't catch it," etc. Obviously, the leaflet we had given them was still sitting on the pile of paperwork. Eventually, we went away with job contacts for H to apply for, and an interview for a volunteer job at a charity which supports people getting into work.

H completed many applications and while she was waiting for responses, she started her volunteer role. After two weeks she was offered a part-time job working there. It was a job-share and she would do twenty hours. I was a little worried about this as it was two and a half days, and although she was used to twenty-five hours at college, that was spread over five days. Also, doing those hours meant she was unable to make any other claims apart from her DLA. But she was determined, and it was the best thing for her.

She was always tired by Wednesday afternoon, but after a rest on Thursday, she enjoyed Friday, Saturday and Sunday. It also meant that the man she job-shared with could cover Wednesday mornings and she would do a full day the following week, to enable her to visit her hospital clinics in London which were on a Wednesday.

She had a brilliant relationship with her job-share man and the rest of the team. Her IT skills enabled her to help others, and she just loved spreadsheets. H worked at this company for five years until the Swindon office closed down and they were all made redundant.

During that time, H had her twenty-first birthday which was also at the same time as Mum/Nan's ninetieth birthday. We held a party at home, and friends and relatives came from all over the country: Lancashire; the Midlands; as well as those closer by.

By then Mum was living in a flat near to us. The party was held in the afternoon and went on into the evening. By 5.00 pm, Mum was tired and her lovely friends Julie and Simon took her home in their convertible car, with the roof down, and Mum sitting there like the queen. It will always be a wonderful memory.

The party continued and when it was winding down at about

10.00 pm, I sent Carly and H out to take down the banners which I had put up on the washing line. The washing line had a pulley mechanism which meant the banners were high up. After about half an hour, they returned and asked for a step ladder to get the banners down. In all her twenty-one years H had not realised that the washing line had a pulley system. They both blamed it on the amount of booze they had consumed – really!

After her redundancy we had to go back to the Job Centre, and they quickly found her a job at the local council where she worked for two years. The department she was in was reorganised, and so she was moved to the Special Needs Department. On her first day one of the team, informed her that she knew me because I was a SENDCo. When H came home and told me, I didn't react in any way, this particular person and I had had dealings at different times, some good, some bad.

The following day, she was given her tasks, which involved filing, computer work, filling in forms and typing letters. She asked for a reasonable adjustment, that someone could get the daily folders out of the filing cabinet (about half a dozen each day), and after she had filed the paperwork, could put them back for her.

Although there were many obstacles she had overcome and learned to do with "dodgy" fingers (H's words), opening filing cabinets and getting files out was not only difficult but the files could be quite sharp. The member of staff I knew suggested that if she was unable to do the job, then maybe she should go home and ask me if it was the right job for her! I was livid and sent an email to the Chief Education Officer, suggesting that a

SEN department should be proactive in encouraging inclusion. I'm still waiting for a reply!

Fortunately, the lovely lady who had placed her at the council found another position for her, where she stayed until it became obvious that work was becoming too much for her. So, after working for eight years, we went back to the Job Centre to claim the ESA benefit.

It took a while to convince the member of staff that she was unable to work. He thought it was a good idea to see under her dressed wounds to make sure she wasn't lying. I understand their need to be cautious, but really? However, as luck would have it, I had some photos on my phone of her open wounds which I had taken to show at St Thomas' Hospital. He went a very funny colour and said that he didn't need to see any more. ESA granted.

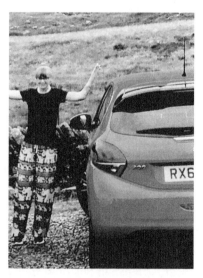

H and her independence. Loved her cars.

# 11

# Media and fundraising

H had always been a great supporter of DEBRA and was always willing to undertake publicity for them. When she was small, it was quite easy to do any local, national or DEBRA interviews for any of the media. There was a period of time, in her teenage years when she was less enthusiastic, at that age, her self-esteem was often challenging and so she only selected to do those that she was confident with. Later on, as a young adult, H was more confident, and keen to raise the profile of EB, and did many interviews, again locally and nationally.

One I remember particularly was for The Mirror, where she explained the day-to-day challenges of living with EB, but at the same time put a positive spin on it with comments like: "There are people worse off than me", and "We have to get on with it!" That's why I am so proud of her. The cameraman wanted a video of her driving her car, so he squatted in the well of the car to film her, I'm sure that was probably illegal, and then a video of me piercing a blister, luckily, we had one to pierce.

We also took part in the "Fight EB" campaign which was a

great success. I always remember Jonny Kennedy's documentary, how brave he was and how inspiring. In the course of being a DEBRA member, I have been amazed at the true grit of many of the RDEB sufferers, especially the older ones, as they see it as something they have to get on with, and this often helps them to keep a positive attitude. I remember one of H's close friends who had RDEB told me that the more negative thoughts you have, the more it drags you down, the whole glass half full/half empty quote. Another RDEB sufferer who died in his early adulthood, also was extremely articulate in explaining the day-to-day trauma of living with his condition but put a positive spin on what he could achieve and how he managed it.

The DEBRA conferences we attended always enabled me to meet up with these special people and also find out about the latest research and medical advances. The first conference I attended was when H was just under a year old. At that time and for the next few years she came along on the trips, usually staying with my mum, while I and my friends attended the conference. The first one was when I met two mums who had children aged two and four with RDEB. They were great supporters and advocates of DEBRA and were behind Princess Diana's coffin going to the funeral. For a short period, Diana was our patron. The parents became friends and I value their support. Sadly, neither of these young people are still with us.

Later on, when we attended conferences both H and I were asked to talk about our experiences, and on another occasion at the retail conference. This was great, as we were meeting the wonderful people who run the DEBRA shops. I have to say that the day ended well for H, as she and a Trustee ended up in the bar drinking "Baby Guinness". Amazingly she didn't have a hangover. In fact, the only time she ever had a hangover was drinking gin with Kevin and she never drank it again.

My main regret is to do with H's boyfriends. She had a few, many didn't last long, but one that she was keen on came to the house on several occasions. She always wanted him to stay, but my fear centred around the physical side of their relationship. My protective instinct overruled my reasoning that young people need to experience that intimacy. I have recently seen posts by the EB community talking about intimacy, intercourse, and sex in general. This is definitely a conversation that requires exploration. I'm sure H shared her thoughts about this and other subjects with her friends, as there are conversations that you feel more at ease discussing with friends than with your mother. I encouraged her to talk to the psychologist when it was offered at our visits to Tommy's for clinic, but she always refused and would say: "I have my friends".

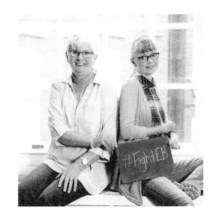

Mum and daughter - Fight EB campaign.

12

Hospital stays

It's very difficult to put H's hospital stays within the body of this text, as they occurred at different periods of her life. I have already mentioned the gastrostomy button insert and the eighteen months of dealing with the eye infection and the events following that. She also had several oesophageal dilatations. In layman's terms, this involved a swallow to see where the restriction was occurring, and then a type of balloon was inserted and slowly pumped up to stretch the oesophagus.

Obviously, this was not without its risks. But after the first two, I think we both got used to it. She had her first one at around eight years old and then regularly every three to four years. It was "fun" when we were at St Thomas', as the ward was on the twelfth floor, overlooking the Houses of Parliament. When bored we could see how much time MPs were in the glass refectory on the side of the building.

I always stayed with H on a mattress next to her bed, until she was in her twenties and then, once she was comfortable, I had a room at the patient/family accommodation next to the hospital. Those people visiting London and excited by listening to Big Ben need to spend time at the hospital overnight, hearing it chime every hour. Double glazing doesn't stop the noise.

H never liked the hospital food and so I used to go to the shops downstairs and get her a tea, caramel latte or ice cream, and once she was feeling better, a toasted sandwich. If we had a long stay, the hospital began to feel like home, the lovely ladies who issued the parking permits, the little man who played the piano, badly! The porters and staff who we knew and would chat with. It never ceased to amaze me, that despite the hospital being so large, there was always someone you knew.

Our dentist was also there and H loved seeing him, particularly when he used to coat her teeth to try and make them stronger. H always referred to it as coating her teeth in Ronseal, I guess teeth are a bit like fence panels. At one point she had a wisdom tooth extracted, amazing that she had wisdom! The team were great in organising this so that it was done at the same time as one of her operations.

H always coped with the idea of operations, but the actual recovery was a different matter. She was always very sick and when she'd had a dilatation this wasn't good. So, when one of the anaesthetists suggested Propofol, H was willing to try anything. From that time onwards she was still sick, but nowhere near as bad as before. On the first occasion after the Propofol, she came around shouting very loudly and declaring love for the anaesthetist. Worst still, because she felt so good, she questioned the porter on his ability to drive a bed, and whether he had training and had to pass a test. By the time we got back to the ward on the twelfth floor, I was completely embarrassed, but George took it in his stride. The volume with which she repeatedly said his name meant that the whole of the hospital knew his name. She did redeem herself by praising him, thanking him and telling him that he was a good driver.

If we had to stay in the hospital for any length of time, or at the patients' accommodation, we always tried to do something. Usually, it was a nice meal at a local Italian restaurant where they got used to us and allowed us to sit in the bar rather than fight our way through the restaurant. H always had the same pasta dish and they were kind enough to make it with only a little pasta, but a great deal of sauce. The London Eye was another favourite activity and a walk along the South Bank.

When we were at GOSH, it was easy to wander down to Oxford Street and look at the shops, always a favourite activity of ours. At St Thomas' I tried to instil some culture. We went to the Imperial War Museum. H showed little interest until we went to see the Holocaust Exhibition. She was fascinated by the model of Auschwitz and asked all sorts of questions of the guide. She even read a couple of books about it afterwards. I decided on another bit of culture, The Tate. There was a Turner exhibition I wanted to see, and so we walked around that and other exhibitions with me chatting all the time, I was suddenly aware that I was getting no response. She was fast asleep in her chair. I didn't suggest it again.

Many of the EB families have a lot more operations and some less. However, they all take it in their stride and just get on with life.

I think the only treatment that H refused to have was the second dose of collagen inserted into her knee. At birth H's leg was badly damaged and was always smaller than the other leg and therefore less effective. It was suggested that collagen treatment would "pump" out the knee and make the leg stronger. H dealt with pain very well but the collagen injection was too much, so she decided not to have the second dose. However, she enjoyed telling people that she'd had a collagen injection, and waiting for people to peer at her face trying to work out where she'd had the injection.

H, like all RDEB sufferers, had many scans and X-rays.

The one that was most frequent was the Dexa scan to look at bone density. H always managed to fall asleep when having scans, I guess she just got used to them. Each week she had Risedronate which had to be taken two hours after eating, then sit up and wait another two hours before eating again, and so it took four hours in all.

H wasn't usually too bothered about food times, but on a Sunday, which is when she took her medicine, she couldn't wait for the time to be up, so that she could have her Sunday roast. It's amazing how you want something when you can't have it. Watching her insert the medicine through her gastrostomy peg was interesting, she pulled the plunger on the syringe using her teeth, sorry dentist, inserted it into the peg/button and then pressed the plunger with her chin to empty the medicine into her body. She did this with all her morning and night medicines unless she was very tired and then I would do it. Where there's a will, there's a way.

Our hospital visits later often coincided with another EB young lady. H and she seemed to mirror their treatments. An amazing and independent lady, who was not going to let her EB stop her from doing what she wanted. H and she became friends, and I know H was impressed by what she had achieved in her life.

Friends and family were always keen to know how H had faired at her hospital appointments. Often on the way home if I was driving, she would send full texts to a variety of people, usually ending with one of her sayings, that at the end of a tiring hospital visit, she would be having a "long horizontal life pause" i.e., sleep. H always had a lot of amusing sayings. Carly and she were always going to "figure things out". If I was on the laptop and made a mistake, my usual reaction was to press every button going, H always said: "Mum, step away from the laptop" while she sorted it out! Her EB nurse was always referred to as "My Jane". Carly and H were always "the dream team" when they were together, they lived off pasta and chocolate oranges (one of her five a day). When faced with adversity she always said: "God loves a trier" (ironic considering she didn't believe). H referred to swear words, of which she used quite a few, as "sentence enhancers"; and her all-time mantra was: "She believed she could, so she did."

But my all-time favourite quote from New Year was when she said to her friends: "Don't expect any New Year's resolutions from me, I intend on staying the same awkward, sarcastic, foul-mouthed delight you've all come to know and love."

The only two words she really hated were "moist" and "penetrate", if I really wanted to upset her, I would see how many times I could include them in a conversation!

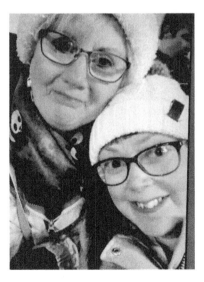

December trip to one of the many Christmas markets.

# 13

# The dreaded C word

In the Spring of 2015 H had a lump appear on her hand. We went up to our usual clinic appointment and a biopsy was carried out. I was due to go on holiday the following week and Carly was, as usual, coming to stay. We were told that the result would take two to three weeks and so the girls persuaded me to go ahead with my holiday and that they all had it under control.

Reluctantly, I left for my tour of Route 66. We had just stopped for lunch at McDonald's on the way to Amarillo, three days before the end of the tour, when I received a phone call from Carly saying the results showed cancer and that H would need an operation. H was obviously devasted, as was I. Carly said they were going to the hospital in two days to speak to the consultant and not to come home. I was with a group of strangers, but they were lovely, the tour guide said that even if I got a flight from Amarillo to LA, it would take about two days to get home and so I continued the tour. The rest of the tour was a blur.

The girls went to the hospital and picked me up from the

airport the next day. I have never been so relieved to be home. Between them, they were very calm and had a plan, they were such stars. H had her operation on June 1$^{st}$ and both Carly and Claire came to visit. The operation went well and she had a skin graft. We got home to a sign on my shopping list whiteboard in the kitchen from Carly which said: "Kicking Cancer's Butt, Yooo Hooo! Big Summer Blow Out. Welcome Home! Dinner's in the fridge."

We went back to dressing the hand and arm like a teddy arm, and a very neat rectangle of skin taken from the right thigh, which once healed, H rubbed bio-oil onto, and the scar all but disappeared.

Even though she was right-handed she made a good attempt at dressing herself and was insistent that she could drive left-handed, until I pointed out that the peg was on the right. But within weeks of the operation she was driving again, back at work and back to her annoying self! I couldn't believe that the wound could heal so well on someone with EB. Our follow-up visit was very positive and the consultant had managed to cut out all the tumour, so there was no need for any follow-up treatment. However, as we left, our honest nurse told us that it might not be the last tumour. I guess we were on such a high that we heard but didn't take it in.

Mum was able to see H's recovery, but sadly she died just before Christmas aged ninety-four. It was devasting for me but more so for H as she adored both her granddad and Nana. At least Mum did not have to live through the next lot of H's cancers, it would have been heartbreaking for her to see H suffer.

~

We had respite for almost a year and then in July 2016, a small lump appeared on the right-hand side of H's neck. Our lovely surgeon operated in October 2016. I was amazed at how large the wound was, considering the lump was very small: a tiny lump with a head on it. It was explained to us to think of it a bit like an iceberg, there is more underneath than on top, and it was essential to have a margin around the area to ensure that all the tumour was taken. This time the skin graft was taken from the left thigh and beautifully lined up, which pleased H with her OCD!

We carefully started to do the dressings and all was going well until one night when we were in bed and H shouted for me. She thought she was sweating, until she realised, she was bleeding from the wound. The blood was everywhere, and for once I didn't know what to do. I phoned 999 and they were amazing. They sent an ambulance which arrived very quickly and they took us straight to A&E.

The doctor who saw us immediately had just transferred from Wales and this was his first shift. I explained H's condition, as by this time she had lost a great deal of blood and was in and out of consciousness. He was completely honest and said that they obviously had covered the condition in his training, but he had never seen anyone with the condition. He quickly found the bleed, which was very tiny, considering there was so much blood, and used a special gauze to stop the bleeding. It worked like magic, and he gave me some to take home, just in case. As I had left home, I had picked up our emergency medical kit and so I was able to redress the rest of her neck, although I left a lot of the dressings which had blood on them, but not enough to make a fuss about.

The doctor and nurses were amazing. I phoned a friend and they took us home. We had only been away from home for a matter of hours, but it seemed like days. H slept like a log. I spent the night in a chair by her bed. EB parents will relate to this. I phoned our nurse in the morning and she organised for us to have an emergency appointment at St Thomas' with our consultant the next day. The news was good in that the bleed had been stopped, but the bad news was that the skin graft had gone. H was outraged, as she said: "Now I have another scar for nothing!" There were no more traumas for a while and her neck began to heal.

In early 2018, we found a lump on H's foot, and because of previous tumours, we were very vigilant and she was seen almost immediately and operated on in February. The op went well, although it was four long hours, but in that time, there is always the preparation and recovery, and we were on our way home after a few days. The protection on her leg was quite large. H had two walking frames provided for her, one for downstairs and one for upstairs. She refused to sleep downstairs and so bottom-shuffled up and down the stairs. We fixed a small basket on both walkers so that she could carry things and H did amazingly well in coping.

I was due to go on a cruise to Iceland with my friend the following week, and was going to cancel, but was assured by H and Carly that they could cope. As the trip was only ten days, I went, and as always, the two existed on pasta, chocolate orange and blinged on rubbish television. I was back in time to take H to the hospital for her check-up. As it was quite difficult to get H in the car with her leg sticking out, so we decided to go by train from Swindon to Reading, then Reading to Waterloo. It was easy to walk from Waterloo to St Thomas'. We had a brilliant journey, a good check-up and were soon on our way home.

The protection on her leg was off and so she was able to bend her knee again, although I was still very aware of the fragility of her foot, even though it was well-padded. On the journey from Waterloo, we met a lovely lady and her grandson and we chatted until Ascot when we were informed that the train was terminating and that we had to get off and catch the next train to Reading. The train pulled in and everyone got off. The lady and her grandson waited with us for a ramp to be brought. We waited, and waited... The driver left the train and we asked where the assistance was, he said he would send somebody, as there was no guard on the train. Afterwards, I thought about it and wondered what would have happened if there had been an emergency, how would we have got off the train? No wonder the train drivers are concerned about not having guards on trains.

Eventually, a ramp was brought, and we left the train to be faced with a staircase, when I asked for the lift, I was told it was not in use, or he may have said there wasn't one. I can't really remember, as I was by this stage, wondering how we were going to get down the steps and then presumably, back up to get on another train. The lovely lady came to my rescue. She reminded me of Hyacinth Bucket (Bouquet), in the nicest possible way. From the top of the steps, she yelled: "I need some strong men to lift this wheelchair". Some of the passengers from the train dropped their bags, came back up the staircase and lifted the chair down about twelve steps, with me shouting: "Be careful, she's just had an operation."

The men were wonderful and very careful. We got to the bottom of the stairs and I asked where we had to go, hoping if it was up another set of stairs then the men would be up for helping again. The station staff informed us that we could go back up to the train that we had just vacated as it was able to go on to Reading. My lovely "Mrs Bouquet", said absolutely not, get her a taxi to Reading. I think the staff decided that she was not to be argued with and did as she asked. I never did get her name, but what an amazing lady, assertive definitely.

The taxi took us to Reading and we caught the train to Swindon. Arriving at Swindon we waited for the ramp. And waited... I could see the ramp and was tempted to get off the train and do it myself. It was the same type of ramp that I had to use to get the electric wheelchair into my car before we had a hoist fitted. Eventually, a man arrived, Reading staff had not notified Swindon staff that a ramp was required, which is what they are supposed to do. I told him that I was thinking of doing it myself, to which he replied in a broad Swindon accent: "You can't do that, it's health and safety". Mmm, it's alright to leave someone on a train, but not allow anyone to move a ramp!

The fourth cancer was in a similar place to the second one, on H's neck. This one was slightly higher and into the hair line and so it necessitated cutting and shaving the hair on her neck. H having long hair meant that her ponytail would cover the dressings once the operation was carried out. This was done in late 2018 by our usual wonderful surgeon. All went well although it was a long operation and I drank vast quantities of tea and even went to the Faith Room. I'm not sure why but I suspect it gave me some peace as it was very quiet. The skin graft was taken from the other side of her right leg, which upset H, as now she was uneven with two on one leg and one on the other. Not good for her OCD. Thinking back, I'm guessing that there wasn't one on the foot, although I really can't remember.

We felt we were in a routine of cancers every year. I spoke

with one of the EB friends and he told me that he had fifteen over a period of time. I guess that was why we became accepting of them. During this time, I remember listening to an interview by another EB sufferer, who said cancer would eventually kill him. I thought he was being rather negative, but guess what? It did.

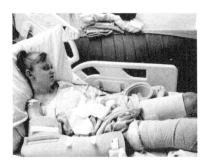

The dreaded C word. H not impressed having her photo taken.

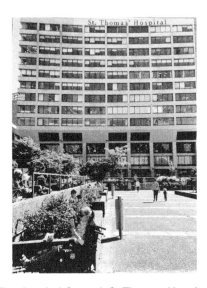

The dreaded C word. St Thomas Hospital.

# 14

# The final cancer 2019

In late 2018 we went up to London for H's six monthly MOT. Just prior to our visit, we noticed a small lump on the front of her left shoulder, which we asked our EB consultant to check out. We enjoyed our clinic visit as usual because it was just before Christmas and so we enjoyed the lights, a walk along the South Bank and a meal at our favourite restaurant. I vaguely remember the consultant saying that she thought this tumour looked different from the rest, but it was Christmas and so I put it to the back of my mind.

We returned in January for the results which were not good. The cancer was terminal, and there was no treatment. I don't think either of us really took it in, as I remember the consultant saying: "Do you understand?" Anyone who has not experienced this kind of statement cannot understand the numbness and empty feeling you experience in your gut. We didn't ask any questions and the journey home was silent, where we usually chatted constantly.

H fell asleep at one point; I think it was from sheer emotional exhaustion. I was left with my thoughts and the tears fell. I had time to pull myself together before she woke, I was determined that we would approach this as we approached all traumas, with a positive attitude, as best we could. Amazingly, she awoke with the same attitude, saying she was going to make the best of whatever time she had left. The text she sent that day as always, must have been very difficult to write and she later put one on Facebook. Despite the devasting news she managed to put her own positive, humorous spin on it.

The next week we occasionally avoided the subject, but when we did talk, it was mostly questions that neither of us was able to answer. Our lovely EB nurses, Jane and Caroline, came down to see us and organised for the doctor from our GP surgery to come at the same time. While the doctor was there, the talk was mostly about H's needs in terms of pain relief and support. The doctor was lovely and it meant that we had a named contact at the surgery. We also discussed the 'Do Not Resuscitate' paperwork, not called that but I can't remember the name, and it will always be the label I will remember it by as we did one for both Mum and Dad. After discussion, H signed it as I felt the tears well up, but I tried to stay controlled.

Once all the nurses had everything in place, the doctor left and we had time for the discussions. How long? What will happen? I was shocked when they both thought it would be a matter of months, I thought we had much longer.

When they answered the second question, I was really numb. They thought her death would be from a traumatic bleed. The tumour by this stage had broken through the skin and looked like a moon landscape. H named it "Lancelot", as you would! My imagination ran wild and after experiencing the bleed on the back of her neck when she had a previous cancer, I could only imagine what this would be like and when would it happen?

One of our EB nurses had been a palliative care nurse in

her previous career, so was able to lead the conversation towards what we should be thinking about. She suggested that H wrote a bucket list of things she wanted to do. Perhaps also to think about what her funeral would be like. I wasn't sure how to deal with that. By the time they left, we were laughing and reminiscing on some of H's more memorable stories, events and sayings. They were both marvellous and found time to support us and be available from then on, with always at least one of them phoning us regularly. I don't think I realised how much work they put in, which made dealing with day-to-day issues so much easier. They also organised for the local cancer nurse to visit, who was very nice, but in the end, although we had her number, H didn't feel she needed them.

About this time, we were contacted by our lovely friend from DEBRA. We had known her for many years and given permission via our EB nurses, for her to be told about H's prognosis. She offered any support we needed from DEBRA, which was gratefully received.

H set about writing her bucket list:

1. A trip to Disney, Paris, with myself and the girls
2. Theatre trip to see *Hamilton* (her friend was starring in it and she wanted to see him)
3. To attend Carly's 30th birthday party in March which was to have a Disney theme, and she was determined to be a dalmatian.
4. To have a tattoo
5. A photographic session to capture photos of her friends.
6. Visit the New Forest, a place we had always been meaning to go to but never got around to. She wanted to see the New Forest Ponies.
7. To attend Sarah and Tom's wedding.

8. One last Olly Murs concert.
9. To be godmother to Sabrina's baby, due in May.
10. Go to Longleat Balloon Festival. We had been to the Bristol one, but she loved Longleat, and although we had been for the lights, never the Balloon Festival.
11. Celebrating my birthday and 50 years of friendship with Boz, which involved cream tea and tapas.
12. Christmas celebrations: pantomime, Christmas markets and Christmas lights.
13. To do a parachute jump or zip wire!

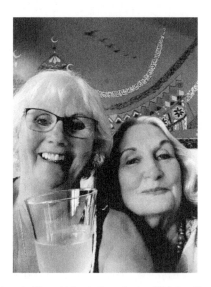

The lovely Boz. H took the photo. Celebrating my birthday.

Being told it was only going to be months, I thought that some of those she selected later in the year were not likely to happen. H had the determination that she would make it!

The next organisation was funeral planning, this was made so much easier by Carly's help. We got a takeaway and sat down to plan. Instead of being a sombre occasion, it turned into one filled with tears of laughter. H had complete control over the planning, and apart from being allowed to select the flowers, because as we know, H didn't realise sweet peas were flowers, everything was what she wanted. Thank goodness for Carly who kept the whole proceedings very light. In fact, Nik, Sabrina and Claire all managed to keep her spirits up, although I suspect H and the girls shared tears, which I know she couldn't do with me, as I was hanging on by a thread. I know my friends found it difficult, all of us being older, there is an unfairness of somebody so young facing death.

And so, the bucket list started.

We had to go to St Thomas' Hospital in February, and so Waylon very kindly organised for us to go and see *Hamilton* while we were there. As the theatre wasn't too far from the hospital, we walked there, finding a lovely restaurant on the way, which of course happened to be an Italian one, had a lovely meal and set off for the theatre. We were greeted and seated. We had brilliant seats, which were easily accessible at the end of the row at the front. The musical was amazing and we were blown away by the cast and the complexity of the dialogue. At the end of the performance, we were collected and taken backstage to meet the cast. They were all so kind and it was so wonderful to see Waylon again. We caught a taxi back to the hospital and were still buzzing the next day when we went for the appointments and were the envy of all the doctors and nurses, especially when H was bragging about knowing one of the cast members. Thank you, Waylon. First bucket list wish achieved.

February was also Valentine's Day and H, Nik and Carly

spent it together. I still have the video they sent me wishing me Happy Valentine's Day, and H complaining that all her "fat" had gone to her chin.

The next was the trip to Disney. When our lovely nurses visited and H had mentioned it, they suggested going sooner, rather than later. So, we started to plan it for March and immediately hit an obstacle. My usual travel insurance company would not cover us. I turned to DEBRA for help, and they organised everything for us, including the travel insurance. Rather than go to St Pancras Station, Nik said she would drive and go from Ashford on the Eurostar. The trip was straightforward. The hotel was lovely and we set off for the park. We watched the parade and the fireworks and I could see H getting more tired, but so determined to make the most of it. We all had headbands with Mickey Mouse ears from our favourite Disney films. Nik – *Moana*; Carly – *Peter Pan* (of course, the girl who never grew up!); H – *The Lion King*; and I had *Frozen*.

I honestly can't remember much about the trip, as in my mind was still the idea of the "traumatic bleed", and we were abroad. I never said this to the girls, but I guess I must have been very uptight, as on the last evening, H was tired and wanted to sleep, I needed to do her dressings, and so we came to verbal blows. I went downstairs for a drink, and I'm guessing Nik and Carly must have said something to H because we all did her dressings and finished the evening without any more cross words. I think they all enjoyed themselves, albeit with the knowledge of it being the last time that they would all go to Disney. But thank you DEBRA for organising it. Bucket list 2 achieved.

March was also Carly's thirtieth birthday, which surprise, surprise had a Disney theme. Carly was Peter Pan, Nik and H went as Cruella de Vil and a Dalmatian. They all looked amazing. I donned a long dress and went as Wendy (*Peter Pan*). Kevin and Jackie made a wonderful Minnie and Mickey. The evening was amazing and the girls made sure that it was a really fun time for H, even though it was Carly's birthday. Bucket list number 3 ticked off.

Despite the pain becoming more pronounced and lasting much longer, H was determined to carry on with her list. Her pain medication was upped and tweaked to try and keep it under control for the whole day, but there were always a couple of hours in the day when she really struggled. Our attendance at Sarah and Tom's wedding was looking doubtful. But on the morning of the wedding, H was determined to go. "After all," as she said, "I've got a new outfit."

She had bought an amazing multi-coloured jumpsuit, looking rather like Joseph and his multi-coloured coat. It was only a short distance to the wedding, so we did the dressings and set off. What a lovely wedding. It was a wonderful day, with lots of people we hadn't met before, making us so welcome. On the way to the wedding, H and I agreed that we would try and see Sarah and Tom's first dance, but that if she felt in pain we would leave earlier. Not only did she manage the first dance but also was still there chatting at 9.00 pm. It was so good to see her with her friends and happy. It didn't matter that she slept the whole of the following day, she'd had a wonderful day. Bucket list 4 – thank you, Sarah and Tom.

The photographic session took place in the garden on a lovely sunny day. Susan is an amazing photographer as well as being mother to H's godchildren. Susan organised for everyone to wear light-coloured tops, so that we blended well together. Besides Susan and the children, Sabrina, Nik, and Carly were there, in charge of hair and make-up. The photos were amazing, and we even managed to persuade Susan to let Carly use the camera so that we had a photo of Susan. Susan put the photos in an album, as she knows that I like photo albums. A beautiful memory. Bucket list 5 – thank you Susan.

Number 6 on the bucket list happened when we went to the New Forest. It was April but still very cold. H loved the ponies, we went to Beaulieu to see the motor museum, and there she was delighted to stand next to the model of the Stig from *Top Gear*, one of her favourite television programmes and the three-wheeler from *Only Fools and Horses*. My dad worked at Fawley in the '80s, so we went to see where he worked. H was still able to drive at this time and so we drove up to the gates and were then questioned by the security guard as to why we were there. After explaining, we left, H said I hope they don't prosecute you for trespassing, it won't matter to me, I won't be here. Every statement like that, even though said with humour was like a knife in my heart. We had two lovely days in the New Forest but on the third day, H asked to go home as she was in so much pain. Was this going to be the catastrophic bleed?

When we got home, H phoned our nurse and told her that she was struggling with pain. Although we had direct contact with our GP and she was helping to deal with pain management, it was decided to discuss it with the EB specialists. So, we took a trip to Tommy's. They sorted a timetable for meds and patches which they felt would keep the pain under control without periods of the day when the pain would become worse. While we were there, we saw our consultant who talked to us about a new treatment which had been developed in Sweden and it was hoped that it would be licensed in the UK. Not a cure but hopefully an extension of the prognosis. At last, some hope. The pain drug regime that was put in place seemed to help and I could see that the pain was more controlled, although it made her very sleepy.

In May, we got a phone call to say that the drug had been

given a license and that H was named as being able to have the treatment. I suspect it cost a lot of money and so there would have been a discussion as to the pros and cons of H receiving the treatment. For the consultation and then treatment we had to go to Guy's Hospital, the link hospital in the trust. Although we had been to Guy's before for a couple of appointments, we had always gone from Tommy's to Guy's by taxi and then back to Tommy's for more appointments. This time we were going straight to Guy's.

We found out that there were very few car parking spaces, but there was an NCP nearby. H drove for the first consultation and we found the car park easily. After we parked, H found the directions on her phone and it said that it was only 500 m. As we left the car park, I was saying that I couldn't see the hospital, a man leaving the car park at the same time, smiled and pointed to a huge building right next to the Shard. Yes, it was only across the road. I then remembered that when we had been to see the dentist on the twelfth floor, you could see into the Shard.

The consultant was lovely and she explained the treatment and that she would have an infusion of an anti-sickness drug before the treatment and then a flush afterwards. H had a scan to see how large the tumour was. By this time Lancelot was massive, covering the whole of her right shoulder down to the top of her right breast. If that was on the outside, I couldn't imagine what was on the inside. It was agreed that the treatment would be every three weeks. We would stay the night before at the patients' accommodation at Tommy's and drive over each Friday morning for 10 am, have the treatment and then go home.

The treatment began.

For the next seven months, we had regular visits to Guy's, trying to make the most of it, we did something on a Thursday evening as we were staying at Tommy's. South Bank, shopping, cocktails or just wandering. Then on to Guy's in the morning. The staff there were wonderful. The canular was always an issue as H's veins, like many EB people, were tiny with lots of scarring. Eventually, she had a PICC line put in, which took the tension out of canulation each time, but the line had also to be kept clear, so we had the stress of wondering every time I cleared it, whether it would block, she still remembered the gastrostomy when the valve blocked. Having the PICC line was much better than the canulating stress had been.

Blood samples were often drawn the day before the treatment, to check everything was alright. They were often taken by the EB team who knew exactly what to do, and they put in the canular. H had to be careful then, not to knock the canular out of place until it was replaced by the PICC line. It also meant we were ready to go when we got to Guy's. Most of the time the routine went smoothly, although occasionally the flush wouldn't go through and then there was a panic in case it was blocked. After the treatment and the flush at the end, we were free to go. The first couple of visits were stressful, but once we had established a routine things improved, with us often seeing the same patients having their treatment, chatting about television, holidays, and fashion. The nurses shared stories of their lives. It was all perfectly normal for people who were fighting for their lives.

The journey home was always a high point. H drove for the first few visits and then began to find it painful and tiring, so I drove and we sang. Our favourite songs were "When the Going Gets Tough, the Tough Go Shopping" (slight change in words); "And I Would Walk 500 Hundred Miles", head swings, followed by holding the reins for "da dum di dum", and bouncing up and down. It was always interesting to see the reaction of other drivers in the queue. "Baker Street" was my all-time favourite song, just because it annoyed H! I used to hum the instrumental bit as we went past Baker Street on our way to Moorfield but then it always seemed appropriate on the way home from Guy's when H used to say: "It sounds nothing like that, and now I'm going to sleep."

On to number 7 on the bucket list. We went to see *The Lion King* yet again (the fourth time I think) but that was an added extra. The birth of her goddaughter was the bonus in May. H had always been close to Sabrina since she had had her children. In fact, she had a regular evening visit to Sabrina (B) and the children, when H used to take KFC for her and B, Sabrina used to insist the children went to bed after saying "Hi" so that she and H could have a good catch up. H got into the habit of taking extra KFC, so the boys had a second tea and stayed up a little bit later. Poor B trying to install a bedtime routine and H destroying it. I think they also used to play games with guns which fired balls, and poor B was trying to keep H safe.

B met Craig and H and he got on well, so KFC became the five of them! Therefore, when B became pregnant H was so delighted, and when Elaina Anne May was born and B had asked her to be godmother, she was just over the moon to see her. The May part of Elaina's name was not because she was born in May, but because it was H's second name. When Elaina was baptised H was struggling, but determined to be there. Flo was over from Canada, and at the baptism party, we met the nursery nurse who had cared for H in SCUB all those years ago. It's a small world and we had gone full circle.

That June she managed all her birthday celebrations with a variety of people and the usual home get-together, with cake, Pimm's and laughter.

Sadly, we never managed to achieve getting the tattoo, as circumstances were against us. Likewise, there was to be no parachute jump. Kevin attempted to persuade the staff of the Zip Wire in Wales to let her have a go, but they said that she wouldn't be insured. H's usual straightforward response was that she was going to die anyway.

Number 8 on the bucket list – Olly Murs. H had booked tickets to see him earlier in the year, but was poorly and in pain and so unable to go. Step in DEBRA again. They managed to secure tickets for his performance at Gloucester Rugby Ground, so not too far for us to travel. They also achieved a meet and greet with him. Apparently, a friend of DEBRA, had a friend who had a friend who knew Olly Murs' manager. Whoever those people are, thank you very much.

I have never seen somebody so excited. I was dragged along with the usual pair of Nik and Carly. We had brilliant seats at the back, high up and although he was very small on the stage, the screens were directly in our line of vision. Before the concert started, we were taken backstage to meet the man himself. He chatted to the girls and we had lots of photos taken. Despite being tired and a little uncomfortable, H insisted on getting out of her chair for all the photos. After the meeting, I asked her what she thought of him. All she could say was that he was lovely and smelt amazing. Whatever aftershave you use Olly, keep using it.

The concert itself was fantastic, although not a massive fan myself, I could see why he is so popular. The girls sang all the way through the set, and I recorded them singing. I've heard better, but not with so much enthusiasm. Their faces showed it all and the quietness in the car on the way home, and H's lack of voice the next day was testament to how much they enjoyed the evening. Thank you again DEBRA and EB nurses for recognising the importance of this event.

My birthday in July was, as usual, me saying: "No celebration" and H going over the top. There were lots of lovely presents including a plaque with a photo of me holding H on her baptism day, and another of H and I wearing out Disney headbands in Disneyland Paris, earlier in the year. The quote brings tears to my eyes whenever I read it:

"First my mum, forever my friend x."

We went out for a lovely cream tea with Boz, but all the photos showed me with my hand across my chin. I had managed to fall over the green waste recycling bin, in the garden, and had to go to A&E to have it glued as it continued to bleed. I'm sure the bin jumped out in front of me.

The next scan at the hospital showed that some of the smaller tumours were shrinking and that the major one had not grown any more from the first scan, so good news. At the same time the tumour which could be seen on top of the skin, began to go black and start to drop off. Lancelot was renamed Lanceless. The tumour on the outside of the skin at this time was about 10 cm x 8 cm.

H had begun to take her cylindrical cushion, called Lilo, everywhere to support her arm where the tumour was. The photos from my birthday show a smiling H but you can see the underlying pain.

Uncle Dai came down from Scotland in August, bringing Monty the dog with him. Monty sat with H on her settee all the time, did he understand?

In September we achieved bucket list number 9. Boz and I had been friends for fifty years, we met at college when we were sixteen and had been through a great deal in that time. H took us to our local tapas bar, a favourite with H and I and we enjoyed a lovely lunch. H was doing so well in keeping going, I was so proud of her.

I think bucket list number 10 was when I began to realise

how much pain and discomfort she was in, and how much she had slowed down. We went to the Balloon Festival at Longleat. It was one of those beautiful end-of-summer/ autumn days, warm with blue skies. Perfect for watching the balloons take off. We had a programme featuring all the balloons which you could tick off as you saw them. I took a picnic and black tea in H's favourite Disney travel mug. She sat in her chair and I sat in a picnic chair. We spent a few happy hours watching and ticking the balloons off on our programme. She was keen to stay until the evening and watch the night balloon flight, but at about 5.00 pm she put her head on my shoulder and said: "I love you, Mum, I think I've had enough, can we go home?"

We had a trip to London at the beginning of October and as usual, H sent a Whats App message to everyone. It read:

"Hi everyone, Yesterday was really positive. We had the finalised results from the PET CT scan a few weeks ago. It's showing measurable reduction of the size of the tumour from the inside, as well as showing measurable decrease in activity. The lymph node which has stopped working and caused the swelling down the right arm seems to have 'calcified' which means the drug has targeted that and is now partially working, which has reduced the swelling and increased the movement in the arm. It was confirmed yesterday that it is now licensed and I'm receiving it through the NHS. Calcium was normal and so I didn't need the reduction drug. Having had a bad time these last few weeks with pain from the back of the neck, it was suggested that I increase the doses per day of OxyNorm and add a higher dose of Fentanyl patch to the current we use, but I have had sickness since upping the patch so we've reduced it again, to see if the increases and sickness goes over the weekend. If it doesn't, we will speak to the EB team to sort a plan. It was also suggested that the drug was attacking the back of the neck, breaking down layers of skin to try and heal it, therefore some of my pain could be nerve related. We've left Dr P to discuss that kind of pain relief with EB consultant. Obviously, the drug will continue over the next 2 years as mentioned before. But we're still being reminded that it is not a cure, it's for a better quality of life, for longer than we were first told when I was diagnosed. For us the priority is reducing the pain in the back of the neck so that I can go out unlike the last few weeks."

No wonder she was so tired and in so much pain.

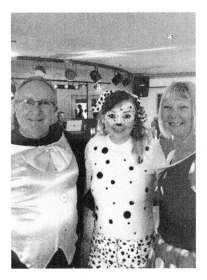

Kevlar, H and AJ- Mickey, Minnie with a Dalmatian
at Carly's party.

We managed to get to Marlborough Mop in October and

have our usual Big Wheel ride, and junk food, but we didn't stay very long. The photo from that shows the fullness in her face and the fixed grin on both our faces. In November, H didn't feel up to our usual fireworks party and so we drove up a hill outside of Swindon and watched the fireworks from there. I did, however, cook the usual jacket potatoes for tea.

Despite all, H used her laptop to plan Christmas presents on a spreadsheet, with a list next to it of where to get the items, mostly online, but occasionally a trip somewhere, or sending me for the Click and Collect. She was so determined for all the presents to be special this year.

Our next visit at the beginning of November showed H's positivity. The Whats App message read:

"Hi Everyone. Had a good couple of days. Dr P is happy with how things are going and seems pleased with the photos of the tumour. I've explained that there are a couple of treatments after Xmas that clash with events I have booked. She was happy to delay treatment or work around things. I'm having a routine ECHO during my next visit. The next PET CT has been pushed back until after Xmas as it's due 19$^{th}$ Dec which is too close to Xmas to be staying around for scans. My calcium level is slightly higher than last time, so as a precaution, I had the reduction drug this morning. My iron level is slightly lower so we'll chat to Jane on Wednesday when she comes for a home visit. Since my last text, I had severe pain across the back of my neck and over my left shoulder. Dr P is convinced that it's inflammation from the drug because it's trying to heal the neck by breaking away 'old skin grafts'. The EB team decided to increase the Fentanyl patch again by 12 micrograms, but as previous, after 4 days of the increase I became really sick which is so frustrating because those days I had the increase were the best pain free days. So, we removed it and the team came up with another drug which I've started on 1.25 ml, it's for nerve pain because they think my nerves are exposed on the back of the neck from where it is trying to 'heal'. This had worked well but not completely eliminated it. Then we had talks about increasing the Fentanyl patch again but only by 6 micrograms. Touchwood – it's working well, I've had no sickness and much better days (and we're on day 8 so past the sickness time!) In mum's words I've "gone from being a miserable cow, to not shutting up". Hoping there's a compliment in there somewhere!!x"

# 15

# Christmas

Bucket list 11

At the end of November, we visited London for H's appointments. We took the opportunity to look at the lights and generally enjoy London at Christmas time. H was on good form and we managed a nice meal and mulled wine. This is her Whats App message from that visit:

"Hi everyone. Sorry it's late, been an interesting day! Yesterday went well. Showed Dr P the tumour as she hasn't seen it properly since before the drug started. She was pleased with the size decrease and healing areas. I have had an antibiotic this week as we swabbed a couple of areas when Jane visited a couple of weeks ago and it came back with 'staph' the usual bug I carry. However, since then there has been a bright 'highlighter green' areas across my body, no pain, no smell, no illness but they decided to swab again as they think it's one of the difficult infections that can only be treated by a limited number of antibiotics. We will get the results and make a plan. Elsewhere, bloods were done, calcium was normal, so I didn't have the reduction drug, my iron was low though. I had my 2 yearly ECHO for the heart yesterday too- yes, they found a heart, I'm surprised too! Arranged Dec's appointment for 19th/20th. Agreed the next progression monitor PET CT will be done in Jan and potentially more iron boost (depending on Dec's blood results) so we will Wed – Fri for that to get it all done. As for today.....a little delay because the staff nurse and matron were in disagreement with Dr P about the iron boost today in the cancer centre as it's usually done in haematology unit. It was done eventually. As for coming home, we were incredibly lucky (especially now we've heard the full extent of the situation today). We got to our car at 1.55 and it all kicked off a few minutes later. We got through (very slowly in huge queues) before all of the closures. First thing we knew was when we saw 30+ police vehicles and police officers were escorting young kids out of school, away from it all. Mum did amazingly dodging flying unmarked police cars coming at us. Got home at 5.30 x."

When we heard the full extent of what happened, H said: "Those people who were stabbed and died, never got a chance to say goodbye to their loved ones. How sad is that?"

The beginning of December saw us doing our usual Christmas activities.

We started with our usual trip to the garden centre to see

the reindeer and buy a Christmas decoration for the tree. Each year we bought at least one, which made our tree a memory tree rather than a trendy one. Usually, we went out with Lorraine to buy our real trees but this year we couldn't find a date which suited all of us, so H and I went alone and finished off with her usual Costa, a Christmas-flavoured one of course, and a cake.

Next was Gloucester Quay Christmas market. When buying chocolate-covered marshmallows; dark chocolate with orange or caramel were H's favourite. We always had to buy twelve as it was cheaper than individually, according to H. We managed to find her a lovely silver bracelet with a heart on it and an adjustable band. For EB people, whose hands are restricted, bracelets are one of those things which easily slip off. Child-sized bracelets are just a bit tight on the wrist of an adult and adult ones just slip off without the expanse of the hand to keep them on.

The Christmas lights, usually at Longleat or Blenheim, were always a favourite. But this time we went to Sudeley Castle after H had researched the access etc. The evening we selected must have been one of the wettest in December. Carly came with us and the journey there was a nightmare. Roads were flooded and the sat nav took us through shortcuts, one of which was a ford. I told the girls to tuck their feet up in case we got flooded. I think I hit the ford rather fast, but I was scared I would get stuck. Needless to say, the journey home was by main roads, the long way round. The lights were lovely, but the disabled access was not quite as good as I had hoped, not helped by the rain. In some parts, it was quite dark which is difficult with a wheelchair and Carly with her dodgy vision, but enjoyable.

We managed our pre-Christmas dinner at a favourite

restaurant with Jackie and Kevin, although we finished early as
H was tired.

I think the most fun we had was going to the pantomime in
Bath to see *Beauty and the Beast* at the Theatre Royal. Getting
a taxi to the station and then the train meant a very relaxing
time without worrying about parking. H had booked matinee
tickets and we had a box for disabled patrons. I bought her a
light-up rose, which she was thrilled with, once a child, always
a child. After the theatre, we went to a lovely restaurant near
the station and had paella and sangria. Although I ate most of
the paella and drank nearly all the sangria. The journey home
was quick, but not fast enough for H to stay awake. I think we
got home at around 8.30 pm and H went straight to bed and
slept until 12.00 pm the following day. Despite the long day for
H, I have a wonderful memory of her laughing at the silly jokes
at the theatre, and singing along to the songs.

Our trip to London for treatment was just before
Christmas on the 20th, and H was not feeling too good after a
fall out of bed, so we bought a meal for two from M&S and just
went to appointments at Tommy's and Guy's. H's message to all
read:

"Hello, well it's been an eventful couple of days. I
epically fell out of bed at 1.00 am on Thursday
morning (I fell asleep sat up- don't ask). Ripped my
knee, my hand, smashed my head (which has ripped
too), ripped my ear, smacked my tumour (and ripped
skin near it), bit my lip and seem to have bruised my
chest, arms and the bottom of my back on the inside.
Poor mum had the rudest and bloodiest wake up call
ever! I'm sorry to anyone who lives near and thought
someone was being murdered – just me being
dramatic! We were debating cancelling London but it

had to be done as next week is still holidays and the first week of January would be silly as we are due back on the 9<sup>th</sup>/10<sup>th</sup> of January. So we didn't have any option. I'm better than I was, just feeling battered, bruised and have a little less skin in places! Anyway, yesterday went well doctor felt calcium drug wasn't needed, my iron is still low so probably have to have the drug to help next time and happy to carry on as we are. Discussions after Christmas will happen about the result pf the PET CT progression scan I'm having on 9<sup>th</sup> Jan. There's talk about going every 4 weeks. Writing this as I'm finishing off the drip and should be heading home in about an hour. Wish us luck for the M4 then our Christmas STARTS!! If I don't speak to you before, have a very happy Christmas! x"

While we were at the hospital H had swabs, which showed she had an infection, and therefore a discussion about antibiotics followed. It was decided on a short course, but as usual, H negotiated the type so that she could have a drink over Christmas. The journey home was fine and we sang Christmas songs and listened to Christmas music, such as Chris Rea's "Driving Home for Christmas", and then H fell asleep.

Christmas Eve was our usual Christmas dinner. H wasn't keen on turkey and so we always had chicken, she especially liked the chicken skin which she savoured and ate very slowly. Her favourite vegetables: courgettes, mushrooms, broccoli and carrots (for colour!). All cooked until very soft to make them easy to swallow, roast potatoes, small and crispy and Yorkshire puddings, maybe not traditional but essential for H so that lashings of gravy made them nice and soft. No Christmas pudding for H, she wanted profiteroles, or tiramisu instead.

Christmas Day was our relaxing day. In previous years we

went out for lunch but after Mum died, we stayed at home and binged on non-traditional foods. H got up late and we did her dressings, lunch was Eggs Royale and then presents. H always had lots of presents, but carefully kept a list of who gave what. I think she probably got this from me, when I did it when she was little and was inclined to rip open presents, losing the gift card in the process. She would text everyone on Boxing Day thanking them, and for those she couldn't text, she would send a thank you letter. Of this, I was very proud - that she always appreciated presents and always said: "Thank you".

I bought H a variety of presents, mostly Disney related but two pairs of lovely earrings, which in hindsight were the most appropriate gifts. One pair was silver filigree and one pair had three coloured gold attached ovals to dangle from her ear.

H thought very carefully about the presents she bought this year, and her friends had scribed mementoes. She bought me a bracelet with the inscription in her handwriting:

"Love you...as big as the world."

How to make someone cry on Christmas Day. She gave me a beautiful card, which she must have struggled to write in, as her right hand was still damaged from the fall, and therefore she had to use her left hand. But she had typed me a letter:

"Mum, Well I'm still here then.... I don't know where to start. I know I say it every year but this year "thank you" really doesn't seem enough. You've been my rock, my pick me up, at times given me tough love (correctly, granted) but most of all you've been my hero. Without you, I know I would be in a completely different position, and not for the better. I'm sorry for being a miserable cow some days, I appreciate I should be grateful for still being here and I forget that sometimes. I'm also sorry for snapping and some of the things I say, I definitely never meant them, I'm lucky to have you. Thank you for always being there, for all you do for me, for taking me out to enjoy things and make memories even though it's a mammoth task and most importantly for never giving up on me. Love you as big as the world. H xxx"

The tears could have floated us away.

How to follow that? Well, we watched *Love Actually* and *Elf.* Our all-time favourites, and snacked on rubbish food all afternoon.

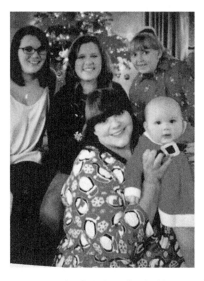

'The usual crew' - Sabrina, Carly, Heather, Nik
and little Elaina - Christmas 2019.

Between Christmas and New Year's Day, we caught up with friends. Usually, on New Year's Eve H would go out with friends and I would often stay at home, as I have never been a lover of New Year. But on this occasion H was tired and so we stayed home and watched television. The major problem was that I recorded all the usual rubbish and so we managed to miss the fireworks going on outside the house but watched them belatedly on the television. So, we actually wished each other a Happy New Year ten minutes after midnight.

# 16

# After Christmas

Our next trip to the hospital was on January 9<sup>th</sup> for scans and we stayed over to see the consultant. Christmas was over and the weather was cold and damp, so we went from appointments back to the patients' accommodation. I bought us a couple of ready meals, did H's dressings - she ate very little - and slept. She was very tired on the way to see the consultant and said very little. She told the consultant that she felt 'rubbish' and was very tearful, so unlike H.

Her text on the way home read:

"Hi everyone. Got home about 2.30, which was really good. An exhausting couple of days but it's all done now. As I've been so tired recently, I had Ferinject (iron infusion) on Wednesday afternoon. We saw a couple of the EB nurses. They gave us a new very diluted bleach spray because they still believe the infection is still hanging around and antibiotics aren't a good idea normally, let alone while I'm on immunotherapy. We also agreed that we would restart my usual iron meds

I'd had for years but had to stop due to sudden intolerance to it last year. Thursday, I had the PET CT and as usual fell asleep! We'll get the results at the next consultation/dose in 3 weeks. We saw Dr H this time, I had a few questions regarding tumour smell which was put down to more tumour dying. Although there were talks with Dr P regarding extending the treatment to every 4 weeks, but at the moment, Dr H says to leave it and we will see what the scan results show. Today was a very early start (6am) but everything went really smoothly. I had the calcium reduction as my calcium was okay but on the 'high' side of okay. Traffic was good, bandages all done and eaten dinner. Looking forward to a very long horizontal life pause (sleep) x."

H even managed to turn the negative into a positive. Feeling poorly but getting on with things!

The following weekend Uncle Dai drove down from Scotland to stay for a few days. Although it was January, his birthday is in February, so we decided to take him out for a treat to the local tapas bar. It was an enjoyable lunch, but not very long because we had left Monty the dog in the car. We then went to Cotton Traders to buy him a shirt, as it's a place he likes to buy from. Unusually, H asked to stay in the car as she was tired from lunch. So, I selected the shirt for Dai's birthday and we went home. Dai cut short his visit as he could see that H was struggling. But I was so glad that he came down.

The next few days, H slept a lot, and in between, we ate all her favourites and watched a lot of rubbish television. The weather was pretty awful and so neither of us really wanted to go out. The girls and Lorraine came as usual for dressings, and H managed to have a laugh with them. The weekend of the 18th/19th came and went quietly, on Monday Carly came for dressings, and on Tuesday, Lorraine came. Tuesday evening was when everything started to happen.

After Lorraine left, H was upstairs in her pjs ready to come downstairs, when I heard a cry go up. Her tumour was bleeding very heavily. I tried to stem the source of the bleeding using the strip of dressing the doctor had given me at A&E on our previous visit, as a just-in-case solution. When this didn't work and I could see H getting paler and paler and less communicative, I phoned 999.

The operator was wonderful and after the initial question which I know they have to ask, although incredibly stressful, she stayed on the phone with me until the ambulance arrived. They were absolutely wonderful and calmed H and me, although, in fairness, H was calmer than me. We explained the situation and by then we had the two paramedics from the ambulance and one from a car which had arrived. After consultation, it was decided that the dressing the doctor had previously given me, should work, and so one of the paramedics took over and distracted us by talking about EB which none of them had ever heard of.

Obviously, because of the position of the tumour, we had to move her body bandage. One of the paramedics was trying to save her dignity by shielding her from everyone else, but she told him not to bother as when you have EB, you are used to flashing your body and boobs around to everyone, and that when you've had a room full of student doctors and the top half of you is naked, then your dignity goes out the window!

H's bedroom although large, seemed very crowded, and it was beginning to be a bit like a party. The paramedic stemmed the bleeding and left us after a couple of hours, satisfied all was well and, after consulting with us, it was decided that hospital admission was not necessary. Although relieved, I was a little apprehensive that the bleed might recur and maybe we should have gone to the hospital, just in case. H was adamant that she wanted to sleep in her own bed.

H looked exhausted, so drink, food and bed seemed the best plan. She had water, followed by a cup of tea and I made her a boiled egg with "soldiers". She was promptly sick after the first mouthful and the tray, egg, etc. slipped to the floor. That was only the second time during her last illness that I lost my temper in front of her, the first being in Disney, all the rest of the time I had managed to walk away and fume elsewhere. I told her she should have gone to hospital and been checked over. She cried and said she was sorry she was such a nuisance, and that when she was gone, I must get on with my life. What a heel I felt. I cleaned her up, and the floor, we had a cuddle, and she fell asleep in my arms. I think perhaps the sickness was from tension and stress. She slept well that night, but I didn't!

The following day H looked much better after a sleep and the bleed seemed to be just a blip in the dying part of the tumour. We had a quiet day and Lorraine came for dressings in the evening, she and H had a lot to catch up on after the previous night's excitement. After she had left, we had a quiet dinner. Wednesday was usually our night out with Jackie but after the previous night, we cancelled it. Television and bed were what we wanted, and this night, I slept very well.

We were due back at the hospital the following week, and so on Thursday, we had planned an early delivery of dressings and meds because we knew that we wouldn't be at home for the delivery on our usual day. Our delivery man from the pharmacy was always cheerful and whistled happily despite having to lift numerous boxes from his car. I spent the rest of the day going up and down stairs, putting boxes away in the medical cupboard and trying to create space. H spent her time on her laptop creating another spreadsheet for all the birthdays she had to buy for in the next few months.

I decided to cook an early dinner and then I would do the dressings after dinner. Dressings were nearly complete when the tumour started to bleed again. Although I managed to get it under some kind of control, H was going in and out of consciousness, and very pale, even for her. I phoned 999 and yet again the lovely operator stayed on the line until a paramedic arrived. This time there was no ambulance and the waiting time, according to the paramedic, was over an hour. He suggested the best thing was to take her by car to A&E as he was concerned about her blood pressure, so he phoned and explained the situation, such that when we arrived at A&E, they would be expecting us.

He suggested that it wasn't a good idea for me to drive, so I phoned Lorraine, who willingly took us up there. She dropped us at the front, and I wheeled H into A&E. The staff were lovely and took us straight through, with several people waiting making comments about jumping the queue! The lady junior doctor said she needed antibiotics and fluids, her blood pressure was so low and she had an infection.

Lorraine joined us and eventually, the nurse got a line in and hooked her up to drips. H was in and out of consciousness but in general seemed pain-free. I eventually persuaded Lorraine to go home, and I dozed in the chair. At about 6.00 pm the doctor came and said there was good news. Her blood pressure had improved, but they were going to admit her to continue the antibiotics and fluids. They were waiting for a bed to become available.

I phoned our lovely nurse, Jane, and she travelled down from her home to be with us. I took the opportunity while she was there with H to go and get clothes, toiletries and dressings as I wasn't sure how long we would be in there. I can't remember how I got home or back, but I just remember getting arms full of things and ramming them into bags. The only thing I really remember was getting her silky pjs, if she couldn't have her satin sheets, at least she'd have her slippery pjs, always easy to get in and out of bed.

When I got back, Jane said that she had been calling for me. H opened her eyes and said: "I love you, Mum, I don't want to die." And I responded with a stupid comment: "I love you, I don't want you to die." That was the last, most coherent statement she made.

A nurse arrived and said the doctor wanted to see me. I followed the nurse and went into his office. I can't remember his name but guess from his suit that he was a senior doctor. He didn't waste any preliminaries, just said: "You do know she's dying?" My first reaction was to respond that we knew it was terminal, but he responded with "She's dying now, her organs are shutting down, she has sepsis." At least I was in no doubt about the outcome of this visit to the hospital. I didn't cry, I was just numb.

I returned to Jane and H. By this time H was unconscious again. So, I explained to Jane what the doctor had said, and she wasn't surprised. She stayed with us for another couple of hours during which time a friend's daughter, a nurse at the hospital, came to see us. I didn't recognise her at first, but it was so good to see a friendly face. Carly arrived and we were transferred to a room on a ward on the third floor. A corridor that we had become used to as dermatology outpatients was on the same floor.

# 17

# The last few days.

Later, on Friday afternoon when Carly and I were settled with H in her room, our friends began to arrive; Boz, Nik and Sabrina. Others asked if they could visit on Saturday. The ward staff were wonderful and didn't seem to mind the comings and goings, even beyond visiting hours. I'm guessing they knew the outcome, although I was still in denial.

Once the others left, Carly and I settled down on our mattresses on either side of H's bed. Occasionally, H would sit up, with a strange look on her face and obviously in pain. At one point she sat up and seemed to smile when I told her I loved her and to lie down and relax. Carly said she was smiling at my voice, but I don't know. We would settle her back down again and she would sleep for an hour or so before sitting up again. In the morning the staff offered us tea and toast which we both accepted. I'm not sure when we had eaten on the previous day.

Saturday morning the girls came back, followed by the ward doctor, who suggested that the fluids and antibiotics were withdrawn. I was reluctant as I still held the hope that the antibiotics would work. I kept remembering a conversation I had had with another RDEB mum whose daughter had sepsis three times, but the last one killed her. Surely this was H's first sepsis, she could recover from this. I phoned Jane and she gently reiterated that this was the end.

I gave my consent for the drips to be detached, but H was still sitting up in pain. The pain management consultant came, and was lovely, prescribing a syringe driver, delivering a steady supply of pain relief. Although her bouts of sitting up reduced, it was still happening. I know on that day I couldn't stand it, if she was going to die, I didn't want her to be in pain. I looked at the pillow as having a different purpose.

In the afternoon friends arrived to see her, and there was almost a party atmosphere in the room, with balloons and chocolates. At one point there were fourteen people in the room. H sat up a couple of times and everyone got excited that she was responding to their visit. Not realising it was pain that made her sit up. Sarah and Tom came in the evening from Reading with the news that they were expecting a baby. As everyone was leaving it struck me that nobody knew this was the end, except the friends who were there when the meds were withdrawn.

The pain relief consultant came to see us, to see how the pain was. She upped the meds which seemed to make her calmer without the sudden sitting up in bed. I told her that it had been awful with so many people, not a calm atmosphere at all. She suggested that her friends probably didn't realise what was happening and that we needed to tell them the facts so that they could come one at a time to say goodbye.

Bless her, Carly messaged everyone and told them the facts and suggested that they returned the next day.

Sunday saw a stream of friends coming to say their goodbyes. Carly and I left them to do so, with me worrying all the time that I may not be there for her final breath. Sarah and Tom came back from Reading so that they could tell her that when the baby was born, she would have Heather as one of her names. A beautiful gesture. Heather and May live on in two beautiful little girls.

Monday was a calmer day. The mattresses were moved and Boz arrived for support, followed by Nik, who had collected more things from the house for us, and Sabrina bearing a tray full of sandwiches; a mini "Earth Mother" following in Boz's footsteps. We had settled into a strange routine of caring for H. All machines had been taken away and so we only saw a nurse every so often. We changed H's sheets because she was wet, but then a nurse came in and catheterised her, so we didn't even have that to do. I tried to change her dressings as H hated not having her dressings changed every day but she stirred and it seemed too painful for her.

Tuesday was a similar day. We included H in our conversations and reminiscences about all sorts of memories, quite a lot of them taking the mickey out of H. Could she hear us?

Wednesday morning Boz arrived, Nik texted Carly to say she wasn't coming and Sabrina arrived with sandwiches at 12.00 pm. Carly wasn't feeling too great and so we put her mattress in the bathroom for her to go and lie down. I was eating one of Sabrina's sandwiches and we were talking food. I was explaining that my mum used to make a pudding which my dad loved, called "Cobweb pudding", it had cooked rhubarb in it, and it was the only time that H ate rhubarb. With that, H took her last breath. I hope she could hear that the last people I was talking about were her beloved grandparents.

Poor Carly, she was there all that time, but not actually for her last breath. Maybe H didn't want her to see that. There was no time to grieve as I had promised her I would change her dressings as soon as she died. She didn't want to be smelly.

Unfortunately, I don't think I had told the others. I went to get the nurse to confirm death and she said that the doctor would have to do it and he was busy. I told her that I needed to change H's dressings. Thank goodness there were four of us. The others didn't make any fuss about doing the dressings. Boz was wonderful as she knew how to move an inert body. Her previous job was as a manager of a care home. Carly was used to the dressings and bless Sabrina, she followed directions. Only afterwards did I realise that Sabrina had not seen H's skin or tumour, it must have been a real shock, but she got on with it.

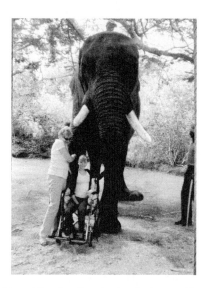

Me, H and Tambo the elephant - happy times in
South Africa.

It was decided only to change the body and neck dressings since the leg and arms were clean as she hadn't moved for several days. That alone took the four of us an hour, moving a body was not easy, especially without the assistance of that body. We put H in a pair of her best silky pjs and tucked her Lilo cushion under her arm. Carly brushed her hair and she looked so peaceful. The doctor came in just before we had finished completing the dressings to confirm death. The nurse had taken off the syringe drive and the catheter. We could feel that rigor mortis was already setting in.

Each of us had individual time to say goodbye and then I cried and cried. My beautiful girl, my best friend, had gone.

The nurse said that a second doctor had to confirm death and then she would be moved to the morgue. I wanted to go with her, but the nurse wasn't sure when they would come. They were keen to get us out of the room, I guess it was needed. We packed up everything and wheeled it down in the wheelchair. Carly's dad came to collect us and they dropped me home at about 5.30 pm. I wandered round and round the house and eventually fell asleep on H's bed, still left how it was the previous Thursday when we went to hospital.

# 18

# Afterwards

The next few days were a fog. I phoned on the Thursday to ask to visit H in the morgue and was told that I was unable to do so until the Friday, as they were waiting for the other doctor to confirm that the death was from expected causes.

I phoned the funeral directors and was lucky enough to get Sabrina's aunty who worked for the Co-op funeral directors. In the past for Mum and Dad, I had used another funeral director but was relieved when Sabrina suggested her aunty as it was good to know that someone who knew her would be taking care of her. She knew H well from family parties and barbecues.

They were unable to collect the body until the Monday, when all the paperwork at the hospital was completed, so I visited H at the morgue on the Friday and then wasn't allowed to go over the weekend as they had a reduced staff and no facilities for visits. I think that was the hardest time, not being able to see my girl.

The visit on the Friday to the morgue was hard but also a time for peace and a chance to have another chat with H. I had to rearrange her Lilo cushion as it was under her head and not her arm. I took a teddy with me to make sure she wasn't lonely; it was one made for her by my friend in St Ives and had a lovely red heart on the jumper.

I made an appointment with the registrar and was pleased when I got there that the registrar was an old friend from the village where I was born. He was so kind and we chatted about my parents and his and that my mum used to babysit him when he was very little. All these things made the pain so much easier to bear. I wasn't prepared for the death certificate in black and white:

a. Severe Sepsis secondary to Pseudomonas Skin Infection; b. Terminal Metastatic Squamous Cell Carcinoma; c. Recessive Dystrophic Epidermolysis Bullosa.

Poor little girl!

On the Monday the funeral director phoned to say they had collected H and I could visit her on the Tuesday. We also organised a time when the director could come and discuss the arrangements with Carly and me.

I then went upstairs and collected all the things to take with me to the funeral director. H wanted a coffin with an elephant on it and wanted it ordered when we planned her funeral. I couldn't face ordering a coffin for someone who was very much alive at that point, so we agreed we would order a drape. A brilliant company responded to my email with ideas and we selected an elephant with a baby in the jungle at sunset, so the surround was a beautiful orange sunset. The edging had a border of small elephants. The drape had been carefully put away since it arrived in April after H had seen it.

I also got the bag that H had put away with her final outfit. Her very favourite *Frozen* silky pjs, her bucket knickers to be cosy and of course her Disney socks. Finally, the letter I had written to her at Christmas which she had read. Words I couldn't say but had written. At a very low moment, H had apologised for being a burden. I had to put this misconception right. She was never a burden, but was the light of my life and my greatest achievement. I wrote all this in a letter, through buckets of tears.

I took her outfit and drape up on Monday, for her to be dressed in and the drape ready for the funeral. I took the letter and also my mum's wedding ring to put in her pyjama pocket – a symbol of both of her grandparents, the ring my dad gave to my mum. As a final thought I took her favourite perfume, "Carolina Herrera 212 VIP".

Tuesday's visit was hard but also very peaceful. Seeing H somewhere safe and hearing that Sabrina's aunty chatted to her was helpful. She would have liked that.

I then visited every day until the Monday before the funeral when it was suggested that maybe it was best to remember her as she was. I already realised that her skin was shrinking showing a thin, not chubby face, and the smell of the perfume was definitely masking the odour.

During that week I got on with the practicalities.

There are a lot of horrible things people have to do when someone dies. Closing bank accounts, sorting direct payments, informing the tax office, etc. H had already told me that she wanted her savings to go to her friends, Carly, Nik and Sabrina and her family as well as Susan and her family. I also knew she would want people to have mementoes of her. The pain of sorting all her prized possessions and asking people what they would like was like a stab in the heart. I kept some of her favourite earrings and all her mementoes from school college and work. One special pair of earrings I decided to put one in her ear and the other I had made into a necklace so that we had something which would join us.

I took her clothes to the DEBRA charity shop but asked for them to be sent to another of the shops, as I was still volunteering at the Swindon shop and did not want to suddenly come across them when doing some sorting. The medical supplies were more difficult. We had a delivery just before H died and so the medical cupboard was full. I really couldn't face taking it back to the pharmacy where I was told it would be destroyed as it was no longer able to be sent out anywhere else. The EB nurses came to my rescue and took away lots of black sacks full of dressings to be sent to support others.

The house began to look very empty.

Sabrina's aunty came to see Carly and I and organise the funeral. We had hardly any decisions to make as H had thought of nearly everything. The flowers were only going to be ones I selected and we were having donations for DEBRA and the World Wildlife Fund - for elephants. I selected an H in white and orange flowers and the card I put on said:

H - Happy
E - Enthusiastic
A - Annoying!
T - Trooper
H - Heroic
E - Engaging
R - Ray of sunshine xxx

The second one was a butterfly with a variety of orange flowers. Then Carly came up with the idea of the Disney logo, this proved quite challenging for the girls at our local flower shop, dyeing flowers black! We had always used the local florist and H always ordered my Mothers' Day flowers and birthday flowers from there, so they knew her very well. In fact, they used to laugh at the way she abandoned the car on double yellow lines to pop in and order the flowers. The flowers were absolutely lovely and they even got me a large sunflower which I put my own tribute on, and was able to put it on top of the coffin on the day of the funeral.

Rob, the man conducting the service, was known to us. We had met him at Sabrina's parents' barbecue on several occasions and he also conducted Jackie's husband (another Rob)'s, funeral. He was lovely and talked us through a difficult plan with compassion, but also humour.

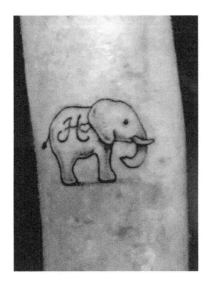

Afterwards. My tattoo. My tribute to my lovely girl.

H had asked for her dad and Uncle Dai to carry the coffin, but Carly and I both decided we would also be honoured to do it. It seemed appropriate for me as I carried H into the world and so I needed to carry her out. Both Carly and I were aware that neither of us knew how to carry a coffin, so we went to the funeral directors to practice. The young man helping us was an old friend of Carly's and so again a direct contact which put us at ease. H would have liked it that we laughed trying to negotiate carrying a coffin with sandbags inside to replicate H's weight.

The days went by getting closer and closer to the funeral. I went onto autopilot, doing all the usual things but without much knowledge of what I was doing. People were wonderful at keeping in touch, but I didn't really want to talk to anyone.

Dai and Monty came and stayed for the funeral. It was so difficult as Monty seemed to be looking for H.

# 19

# The funeral

This poem by Kelly Roper, H liked. I don't know if we used it but it sums up the day.

*Please excuse me for not getting up.*
*Oh dear, if you're hearing this right now,*
*I must have given up the ghost.*
*I hope you can forgive me for being*
*Such a stiff and unwelcoming host.*
*Just talk amongst yourselves my friends,*
*And share a toast or two*
*For I am sure you will remember well*
*How I loved to drink with you.*
*Don't worry about mourning me,*
*I was never easy to offend*
*Feel free to share a story at my expense*
*And we'll have a good laugh at the end.*

It had been suggested that H's funeral took place at the end of the day in a double slot, so it was on Wednesday February

19<sup>th</sup> 2020. I had booked the local pub for the wake and another coincidence was that one of the staff was the daughter of a colleague and friend I had previously worked with. She and her boss were amazing at suggesting how many people we needed to cater for. Carly said that she and H had had a conversation about alcohol, and they had decided that everyone should have a shot of Sambuca, H's favourite. It was her final laugh at me, as she knew I hated Sambuca.

Wednesday morning seemed to go on forever. The hearse arrived, and the car to take us to the funeral. Carly came with me; Dai took his van because of Monty the dog. Suddenly it became real. It's only a couple of miles to the crematorium and when we arrived, I was amazed to see so many people there.

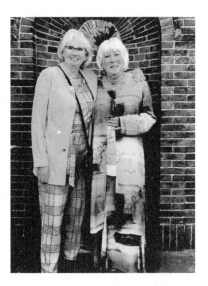

The funeral. I was fine at the funeral until I saw
this wonderful lady, Jane.

At first, I thought they were running late and that some of the people were waiting for the previous funeral. Then I began to recognise faces, the funeral director estimated 250 people were there. The actual chapel did not hold that many, but luckily, they have a waiting area with a screen. There were orange shirts, scarves, ties and I found out afterwards, even orange socks. H would have been so pleased that everyone noted her wishes. I also realised that some of my ex-colleagues and friends were on half term, so I guess they didn't have the problem of getting time off to attend.

My lovely friend from Brighton was there with her daughter and up to that moment I was holding it together. She and I had always been there for each other through many traumas.

Carrying the coffin proved more difficult than I realised, and so two of the staff from the funeral directors helped Carly, Heather's dad, Dai and I to manoeuvre the coffin. They all coped much better than me, as I had completely forgotten about lowering the coffin and sliding it onto the stand. I vaguely remember people directing me.

The sunflower was on my seat, so I placed it on the coffin, so hard to believe my beautiful daughter was in that "box". The drape was to be left on the coffin and cremated alongside H. Cremation was her choice, as she said: "I don't want to be buried, to get cold and for the bugs and worms to get me!"

The order of service, or "programme" as H called it was lovely. The photos were all selected by H and Carly and the actual printing was on card with shadow elephants and trees along the bottom and a light orange hue as the background.

Rob conducted the service beautifully, painting a wonderful picture of H which he had gleaned from Carly and I discussing her with him. The entrance, carrying the coffin, was to the music of the 'Greatest Showman: "This Is Me". She loved the musical and the film. Her favourite line was, "I am brave, I am bruised, I am who I'm meant to be, this is me." She sang it with such vigour even with a pitchless voice.

I thought long and hard about what I was going to say and although she was amazing, she had her moments which I tried to reflect in my piece: "H". Carly did an amazing job, bringing humour and emphasizing the joy their friendship brought to both of them, in her contribution: "Dude". With her talent, she had put together photos of H, family and friends, which was shown while "Hakuna Matata" from *The Lion King* played. I'm guessing H and Carly had more conversations about her funeral after the initial one we had.

H had even chosen her poem: "Please don't cry" (with tears streaming down my face while I am typing this).

> *Please don't cry because I'm gone,*
> *Smile because I carry on.*
> *You'll always be able to find me*
> *In all the little things that you see.*
> *You'll be reminded of the things*
> *That would always make my heart sing;*
> *Maybe a certain song we shared,*
> *Maybe a place when you and I were there.*
> *I'm not in pain anymore and I can walk*
> *When you see me again we'll have a talk,*
> *Because where I am, I am whole –*
> *Shining like a beautiful soul.*
> *Remember my laughter, remember my smile,*
> *Remember my love and my carefree style.*
> *Remember my zeal for living,*
> *Remember my heart that was giving.*
> *Remember my strength and carry it with you.*
> *Remember, I'll always be next to you.*
> *In your heart and in your mind*
> *I'll be there for you to find.*
> *Remember my fire to always pull through,*

*No matter what life tried to do.*
*Remember the twinkle in my eye.*
*Remember me, but please don't cry.*

Of course, we had to have an Olly Murs song: "Dance with Me Tonight" was selected. Followed by "Her Jane" giving a lovely tribute to "My Heather."

Soon it was time for a last goodbye and "I Will Always Love You" by Whitney Houston. All the time H was in the funeral director's, I felt she was close to me, now suddenly she was going. All I really wanted to do was go home and pull the bedclothes over my head.

But, there were people to see. People who had travelled from Cumbria, Nottingham, Cornwall, Lancashire: family, ex-colleagues, H's teachers, friends of mine, friends of Heather's, DEBRA staff, EB families, and people who I hadn't seen for years, who had made the effort to come and say farewell.

I was touched that Simon Weston the president of DEBRA came. He had come to our house when he first became president. H was so in awe of his courage. He was a very kind man who disappeared after the funeral, as he didn't want to take away any of the focus of the reason for being there. I was staggered by people's kindness and generosity- they donated nearly £1000 to Debra and over £600 to WWF - elephants.

Not everyone came to the wake, but there were many there. I can't remember much about it except I read a poem by Spike Milligan which H and I liked:

*Smiling is infectious you catch it like the flu,*
*When someone smiled at me today, I started*
*   smiling too.*
*I walked around the corner and someone saw*
*   me grin,*

*When he smiled, I realised I'd passed it on*
   *to him,*
*I thought about the smile and then realised its*
   *worth,*
*A single smile like mine could travel round the*
   *earth.*
*So, if you feel a smile begin, don't leave it*
   *undetected,*
*Start an epidemic and get the world infected.*

Then we had the Sambuca shots.

Carly had put together a montage of photos and people were encouraged to write around its border. This and a vast number of cards written on the day of the funeral, others which arrived before and after the funeral, letters from friends and professionals have always given me comfort and I read them regularly.

I remember getting home about 6ish, I'm not sure how. Family from the north called in before they went to their hotels. More people called in the next morning and Dai stayed for a few days.

Then I was on my own.

# 20

## Life after H

The paperwork continued, but most of it was done. I had spent time sorting H's personal effects between her death and the funeral, mostly to stop myself from sitting and thinking. People were very kind and phoned or texted me, I think my response was probably quite brief, there was not much to say. The end of February was very hard. I collected H's ashes, it had been agreed that they would be put in one large container and three small ones. The large container was decorated with a beautiful orange sunset over a field of sunflowers. I gave one small container to Carly for her to scatter at Westonbirt where they always went in the autumn to see the lovely coloured leaves, especially the orange ones.

One of the smaller containers I kept in my memory cupboard with a small amount of Leah's ashes, the rest of Leah's ashes I put with H's, so they could be together when they were scattered. I had three tokens with H's ashes made up for me (I always carry her with me), and her godmothers, Jackie and Flo.

It was too early in the year to go to Weymouth, where her

ashes were to be scattered, so that was planned for later in the year. The first weekend in March was beautiful, and weekends were, and still are, very difficult, so, I took myself over to the village with a picnic and the small container of H's ashes. I played "Pooh Sticks" on the bridge, on my own, but with two pieces of bark, leaves or grasses. H won every time. I scattered a few ashes in the river and drove on to Savernake Forest, to the monument, a place where we had lots of picnics with Mum and Dad. I scattered a small amount there and had my picnic.

The following week I felt in control enough to go back to my routine. I went to the DEBRA shop to do my volunteering, had a swim with Lorraine, volunteered at Headway and my History Society. While I was busy there was no time to think, except going back to an empty house every day was something I wasn't used to. This routine continued for a couple of weeks and then the COVID19 lockdown began!

I know everyone says lockdown was difficult for the children but at least they had family around them and social media to keep in touch with friends. People living on their own only had social media. Boz and I kept in close touch, as her family lived some distance away. Thank goodness the weather was good.

I kept myself occupied with painting the rooms in the house and gardening. Sabrina managed to get me some plants for the garden and Nik had given me sunflowers to grow in H's memory. Sabrina did my shopping for me for the first couple of weeks, as Boris Johnson said that the elderly were at risk. Suddenly, I felt elderly which I had never felt before. After, a couple of weeks I ventured to the shops so that I could see other people. I had my lovely neighbours and we chatted over the fence, but even my half an hour walks only allowed us to say "Hello" at a distance to fellow walkers.

In the evenings I made memory cushions, using some of H's

favourite clothes. I sewed together hexagons in the shape of H and the initial of the person I was making it for, and sewed these onto plain cushions. I think I made ten in all, including a memory pillow for myself. I also knitted for Sabrina's children, doing anything to keep my brain and hands occupied.

Towards the end of the first lockdown on my walks, I went to the cemetery to look at Kais' grave as Boz hadn't been there since lockdown and she usually visited him every week. I stopped and chatted across gardens with friends who lived nearby. I was always worried that I might be breaking the rules.

On one occasion I drove to Boz's with a car full of provisions she didn't really need, in case I got stopped, and stood at the wall while she stood on the doorstep and chatted for half an hour, then took the provisions home again! I just needed to see people in the flesh and not on Zoom. It is strange to think that generally, the British public was sticking to the rules while the government had lots of flexibility. I don't want this to be political, but I'm sure lots can relate to it. Thanks Boris!

During lockdown, I was able to email the crematorium and order a plaque to go on a memory vase next to Mum and Dad. I was lucky that the one next to Mum and Dad had become vacant and so they were together:

"Heather Skerry 1990-2020. H- brave superstar.
Hakuna Matata xxxx."

I also ordered a tree for the Skerry family but that had to go into a lottery, as so many people wanted trees at the crematorium, and I had to wait until July for the decision on whether I could have one, and then the tree wouldn't be planted until late autumn. I also had H's name put in the Remembrance Book again, Mum and Dad had theirs recorded on the day of their deaths. I had the symbol of a sunflower and the text saying:

"Skerry, Heather May 1990-2020 – Aged 29 years.
Inspirational, brave and funny. Love you as big as the world xx "This is me" – hakuna matata xx"

Meanwhile, I ordered a plaque for Clevedon Pier to go with the Skerry plaque, Mum's, Dad's and Rob's. This had one of her favourite quotes on it:

'Heather May Skerry 1990-2020. When life gives you a hundred reasons to cry, show life that you have a thousand reasons to smile and laugh. Hakuna Matata xx

Apart from the tree, these were all tributes H and I discussed, it was just up to me to decide on the wording. At least I had something to focus on during lockdown.

Obviously, like everyone, we were restricted until June. When the government realised people were becoming isolated, they introduced the 'bubble', and Jackie and Kevin became my bubble. In June we went to Clevedon to see H's plaque on the pier and polish the other ones while we were there. Burnham on Sea's takeaway of fish and chips had never tasted so good.

Also, in June it would have been H's thirtieth birthday. By this stage, we were allowed to congregate with six people outside. We had Pimm's and snacks in the garden, drank to H and let off balloons. We didn't have to worry about aeroplanes as nothing was flying. Jackie, Kevin, Carly, Nik, Sabrina and I sat and chatted and shared memories. There were only six of us so we were not breaking the rules. My lovely friend Sal made a beautiful tapestry for H's memory, with orange elephants and butterflies, it takes pride of place in my house. She also had cards made of the tapestry that I sent to friends, and the inscription read:

"Dedicated to the memory of Heather May Skerry. A brave and beautiful soul, who would have been 30 on 13<sup>th</sup> June '20."

Original piece was hand dyed, and painted silk, stitched, embellished and appliqued.

After H had died and I was going through her paperwork on the laptop, I found a spreadsheet for Jane, our nurse who was retiring. However, with Covid, Jane had had to postpone her retirement. I knew H had intended putting together one of her special baskets with all sorts of gifts. I was then tasked with completing it. H had left websites where I could access the gifts that she wanted to give her, and very soon I learned how to order online. H had always done it previously and so it was a good learning curve. I was able to complete the task and when we were allowed, I met up with Jane in Bourton-on-the-Water, I gave her the basket, we cried, we walked, and I was able to ask her some of the questions which had been nagging at me.

I had always wondered that if I had insisted on going to hospital on the Tuesday would the outcome have been different? Jane obviously couldn't answer that, but she did say that the treatment was never a cure for H but to give her more time, and that both she and Caroline were surprised that she had a whole year from the diagnosis. We agreed that H was very determined, especially to be there for Christmas!

When we were all allowed to travel again, I managed to see Sal in St Ives, Maxine in Liverpool and Jane in Saundersfoot. But each time it was back to an empty, very clean, house.

I occasionally met people who would ask about H and

hadn't realised that she had died, but I wasn't prepared for a phone call from Direct Payments in May, asking to speak to H. All the other organisations had been really helpful and there were no problems. At first, I didn't know who it was, as the company had a name that I didn't recognise, since I wasn't used to dealing with them. I cautiously asked if I could help and they responded by telling me that she hadn't filled in the tax forms for the last four months, for the people she employed under direct payments. When I said H was dead, there was a deathly hush (excuse the pun). I suggested that their departments talk to each other. People do not realise what a profound effect a comment like that can have on someone who is grieving and doing their best to cope.

Dai came from Scotland to see me in August and we went out for dinner with Kevin and Jackie ("Eat out to help out" - an initiative organised by Rishi Sunak). They had both had tattoos in honour of H, and nearly on the same day. Kevin's is Simba the lion cub with "Hakuna Matata" written underneath, it's tattooed on the inside bend of his arm, so that when he bends his arm and then straightens it, Simba seems to be roaring. Dai's says "Hakuna Matata" in bold writing and coloured in orange. So lovely that both thought of the same idea.

The DEBRA team allowed me to book the caravan at Bowleaze Cove in Weymouth at the beginning of October and so Jackie, Kevin, Nik, Carly and Sabrina came with me to scatter H's ashes. It couldn't have been a worse day, wet and windy. Scattering the ashes was challenging and one of the girls suggested that we keep the rest of the ashes to scatter around the tree in the crematorium when it was planted. We debated as to where to scatter the ashes as we all decided that although H liked the sea, she didn't actually like going in it. In the end, we scattered them on a lovely green area overlooking the sea, but near the car park, ready for visits.

I had been notified that a tree was going to be planted for us, so we had somewhere else to scatter the ashes. After our little ceremony where we scattered the ashes and some orange petals which one of the girls had brought, we went to the arcade and put 2ps in the "Tipping Point" machine. The girls stayed the night in the caravan with me and then went home on Sunday. Jackie and Kevin stayed at the local hotel and we went on Monday to have a cream tea in Portland, another of H's favourite spots and her favourite food. They went home on Monday evening and I stayed until Wednesday, just walking and remembering.

Thank goodness we scattered the ashes then, because we had a further lockdown in December. It didn't have a massive impact on me as I was intending spending Christmas on my own, but I did feel for families who couldn't get together. I replicated the year before when H and I stayed in our matching Christmas pjs and ate Eggs Royale, and watched *Elf* and *Love Actually*. But this time I just cried.

Jackie and Kevin bought me an elephant knitting pattern for Christmas, and so I made one, sewed H's initial on it and put an orange ribbon around its neck. This was the first of a herd of elephants I knitted, I adapted the pattern to be able to make smaller ones and knitted elephants for everyone. It was a great evening filler.

I was informed just before Christmas that the tree was planted and a plaque was in place but with the second lockdown, we had to wait until January to scatter the rest of the ashes. This time Jackie, Rich, Lorraine, Susan, Jackie and Kevin and I did the honours. I think the ruling was back to only six people allowed to gather outside and so we broke the rules. I was delighted with the plaque as it was for Mum, Dad and H and read:

"Super Skerrys"
Reg aged 87 always smiling
May aged 94 kind and caring
Heather May aged 29 funny, inspirational and brave
Loved and missed by me
Loved by many others
"They leave footprints in our hearts"
Xxx Hukuna Matata xxx

The day was beautiful, if cold and difficult to believe that it was a year since H had left us. And what a year it had been.

After the second lockdown was over, I re-evaluated what to do. I decided that the house was too big. Generally, the memories were good but I needed to downsize, especially the garden. With Boz's help, I found a house which just happened to be near to her. The packing up and getting rid of things was hard but it gave me a focus. I eventually moved in September and set about my new project of making the house my own. It only had two bedrooms and so one was mine and the other was H's. On H's bed, there is a beautiful large quilt.

The quilt was made by Flo, started before H died and she sent her many photos, which Flo incorporated. The centre panel is a mother elephant with two babies and an orange sunset. Surrounding this are photos of H from baby to grown-up, with a variety of people with her, some still with us and some who have passed, and around the edge is a frieze of elephants. It was absolutely beautiful. On the back, Flo had embroidered the names of important people in H's life.

In October I completed the last of H's bucket list.

Kevin found me a lovely girl to do a tattoo, I emailed her and said I wanted an elephant with an H on it. I explained what it was for and she was very kind in her response. She asked me to send her a picture of the elephant, which I did, and we fixed a date for the "operation"! I went with great trepidation, but she soon put me at ease. Deciding where to have it was easy, the least painful place, on the front of my lower arm. We chatted about music and she decided that she had Queen music that she would play. We chatted about the fact that lots of people get hooked on having tattoos. I found the actual procedure uncomfortable rather than painful. In the end, I was really happy, but I asked if I could have a small heart put on, which she did and then filled it in with orange. All done. The last question was: "Was I hooked on tattoos?" My response was: "It was as painful as I first thought it would be, but no I definitely wouldn't be having any more."

That was the first of the two remaining bucket list items completed.

The remaining one was a parachute jump or zip wire. I opted for the zip wire and so Kevin booked the one in north Wales. He had already done it once, and so he said he would do it again with me. The DEBRA team again kindly allowed me to book the holiday home in north Wales, and Kevin, Jackie and I went up on the Sunday, ready for the zip wire trip on the Tuesday. We spent Monday in the rain, visiting castles. In the evening Kevin said that the zip may be cancelled due to the weather. I decided that if it was cancelled, then no way could I do it on another day, my stomach was already in knots. But as luck would have it, the next day was dry, if a little overcast.

Kevin and I set off, leaving Jackie in the café. First, we went onto the small wire. I was absolutely terrified. Harness and helmet were put on, I was lying on the table, the table lowered and then I was off. I felt as though I was really close to the trees and rocks, although I know I wasn't, and then the jolt on landing shook my whole body. I told Kevin that I didn't think I could do the other one, he assured me that it wasn't as bad.

We went up to the long zip wire in a Land Rover-type vehicle, that was an experience in itself, being bounced all over the place. The same format followed: harness, helmet, on the table. A member of staff asked me if I was OK, I mumbled something, and Kevin explained why I was doing it, the guy patted me on my helmet and said: "Well done." I remember Kevin saying: "for H," and then we were off, it was amazing! Over the quarry I went, seeing the blue water below, the trees and plants. Travelling so fast (about 100 mph I think), it was over too quickly, and even the landing was smooth. I was so pleased that I didn't give up after the first zip, the second one was just unbelievable. H would have loved it.

We had a lovely meal in the evening and a bottle of wine and raised a glass to H. We had completed her bucket list, noting that she had left me the traumatic things to do.

The girls also had tattoos, each with their own memories.

At the end of 2021 and into 2022, I focused on getting the new house how I wanted it. Dai came down and worked his magic on doing all the things I wanted to be done from my extensive list on A4 paper. I continued my volunteering at the DEBRA shop, which gave me a focus and a meaning. At the end of 2022 and into 2023, I needed a new focus, which is how I came to write this.

Initially, as I said at the beginning, it was for me to remember all the good times and not focus on the last year of H's life. But since starting, I have seen posts from DEBRA asking EB sufferers and their families to share their experiences of living with EB, so I have decided that it may be a useful book for others to read. So at this moment, I think I may pay for it to be published and sell the copies as a fundraiser for DEBRA. Although the latter half is very sad, I'm hopeful that all the fun and things H achieved will override this. As H would say: "She believed she could, so she did".

Now I have completed this, I need to find another focus for my life. RDEB parents will be able to relate to the fact that having an EB child becomes the focus of your life, while one always gets on with life, EB and its associated issues are always there.

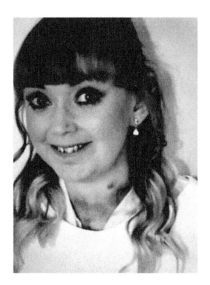

Gorgeous girl.

# Acknowledgements

My few family and friends who support me day in and day out, locally and around the country, for the last three years. Contacting me daily or weekly, messaging or meeting. You know who you are, thank you.

EB medical professionals, not just the wonderful nurses and doctors, but all others supporting sufferers and their families.

DEBRA – for all their support in making life a little bit easier for sufferers and their families.

The amazing DEBRA charity retail shops around the country, but especially the Swindon shop which has done so much to support me in the last three years – Sarah and the volunteers.

Ali and Bob who have no idea what inspiration I got from them, to give me the confidence to write the book.

And finally, my beautiful daughter, who taught me the value of life and how to differentiate between the important things to concern yourself about, and those of no real consequence.

## We Love Memoirs

Join me and other memoir authors and readers in the We Love Memoirs Facebook group, the friendliest group on Facebook. www.facebook.com/groups/welovememoirs/

Printed in Great Britain
by Amazon

25713038R00106